14

A Colour Atlas of
Respiratory Infections

CHAPMAN & HALL MEDICAL ATLAS SERIES

Chapman & Hall's new series of highly illustrated books covers a broad spectrum of topics in clinical medicine and surgery. Each title is unique in that it deals with a specific subject in an authoritative and comprehensive manner.

All titles in the series are up to date and feature substantial amounts of top quality illustrative material, combining colour and black-and-white photographs and often specially developed line artwork.

Slide Atlases are also available for some of the titles in the series.

The amount of supporting text varies: where the illustrations are backed-up by large amounts of integrated text the volume has been called 'A text and atlas' to indicate that it can be used not only as a high quality colour reference source but also as a textbook.

1. **A Colour Atlas of Endovascular Surgery**
   R.A. White and G.H. White
   Also available:
   A Slide Atlas of Endovascular Surgery

2. **A Colour Atlas of Heart Disease**
   G.C. Sutton and K.M. Fox

3. **A Colour Atlas of Breast Histopathology**
   M. Trojani

4. **A Text and Atlas of Strabismus Surgery**
   R. Richards
   Also available:
   A Slide Atlas of Strabismus Surgery

5. **A Text and Atlas of Integrated Colposcopy**
   M.C. Anderson, J.A. Jordon, A.R. Morse and F. Sharp
   Also available:
   A Slide Atlas of Colposcopy

6. **A Text and Atlas of Liver Ultrasound**
   H. Bismuth, F. Kunstlinger and D. Castaing

7. **A Colour Atlas of Nuclear Cardiology**
   M.L. Goris and J. Bretille

8. **A Colour Atlas of Diseases of the Vulva**
   C.M. Ridley, J.D. Oriel and A.J. Robinson

9. **A Colour Atlas of Burn Injuries**
   J.A. Clarke

10. **A Colour Atlas of Medical Entomology**
    N.R.H. Burgess and G.O. Cowan

11. **A Text and Atlas of Arterial Imaging**
    D.M. Cavaye and R.A. White

12. **A Colour Atlas of Respiratory Infections**
    J.T. Macfarlane, R.G. Finch and R.E. Cotton

13. **A Text and Atlas of Paediatric Orofacial Medicine and Pathology**
    R.K. Hall

In preparation

A Text and Atlas of Clinical Retinopathies
P.M. Dodson, E.E. Kritzinger and D.G. Beevers

A Colour Atlas of Retinovascular Disease
S.T.D. Roxburgh, W.M. Haining and E. Rosen

A Colour Atlas of Forensic Medicine
J.K. Mason and A. Usher

A Colour Atlas of Neonatal Pathology
D. de Sa

A Text and Atlas of Breast Cytodiagnosis
P.A. Trott

A Colour Atlas of Respiratory Infections

J.T. Macfarlane, MA, DM, FRCP
Consultant Physician in General and Respiratory Medicine,
City Hospital, and Clinical Teacher, University of Nottingham,
Nottingham, UK

R.G. Finch, FRCP, FRCPath, FFPM
Professor of Infectious Diseases, City Hospital and University of
Nottingham, Nottingham, UK

R.E. Cotton, MD, FRCPath
Emeritus Consultant Histopathologist/Cytopathologist,
City Hospital, and Special Professor in Diagnostic Oncology,
University of Nottingham, Nottingham, UK

CHAPMAN & HALL MEDICAL
London · Glasgow · New York · Tokyo · Melbourne · Madras

Published by Chapman & Hall, 2–6 Boundary Row, London SE1 8HN

Chapman & Hall, 2–6 Boundary Row, London SE1 8HN, UK

Blackie Academic & Professional, Wester Cleddens Road, Bishopbriggs, Glasgow G64 2NZ, UK

Chapman & Hall Japan, Thomson Publishing Japan, Hirakawacho Nemoto Building, 6F, 1-7-11 Hirakawa-cho, Chiyoda-ku, Tokyo 102, Japan

Chapman & Hall Australia, Thomas Nelson Australia, 102 Dodds Street, South Melbourne, Victoria 3205, Australia

Chapman & Hall India, R. Seshadri, 32 Second Main Road, CIT East, Madras 600 035, India

First edition 1993

© 1993 J.T. Macfarlane, R.G. Finch and R.E. Cotton

Typeset in 10/12 Palatino by Keyset Composition, Colchester, Essex
Printed and bound in Hong Kong

ISBN 0 412 38960 6

Contents

Preface

Infections of the respiratory tract are one of the commonest causes of illness that present to doctors both in the community and in hospital and are a major cause of morbidity and mortality in both developed and developing countries. The spectrum of disease is wide, varying from the attack of sinusitis or bronchitis seen by the community-based physician through to complex and sometimes multiple infections in immunocompromised and HIV-infected individuals.

The correct approach to the patient requires a broad overview of the clinical, microbiological and pathological features of the topic and of particular infections. The clinician can only make logical management decisions if he is fully aware of the epidemiology and pathogenesis of infections and how the microbiologist can help him. Similarly, the microbiologist must have a grasp of the situation faced by the clinician.

In this book we have integrated the essential information that the clinician must be aware of with an in-depth look at the microbiological and pathological aspects, both of broad groups of respiratory infections and also of specific pathogens.

We have illustrated points with real case histories to add interest and reality to the text.

The illustrations are fully supported by authoritative text that emphasizes the practical management and will be of value both as a learning aid and for patient management.

The importance of different pathogens varies around the world and there are sections on respiratory infections peculiar to certain geographical areas such as the tropics and North America.

We hope that the book will be of value to trainees in internal and respiratory medicine and infectious diseases as well as laboratory-based microbiologists and pathologists. Paramedical staff such as infection control nurses and microbiology scientific officers will also benefit from the text and colour atlas approach.

We have enjoyed collecting together the many illustrations and have been most grateful for the help of many colleagues who have made this possible and who we acknowledge elsewhere. We hope the reader finds the book enjoyable as well as useful and easy to use.

We dedicate this book to Rosamund, Eunice and Sue for their encouragement and forebearance.

We are most grateful to the following Colleagues who kindly provided figures for use in this Colour Atlas.

Dr D. Baldwin, Nottingham (Figs 10.13, 10.20–10.23)
Dr A. P. Ball, Windygates, Scotland (Fig. 4.67)
Dr C. L. R. Bartlett, Colindale (Fig. 4.2)
Mr P. Bradley, Nottingham (Figs 3.4, 3.8)
Dr E. H. Bossen, Duke University, USA (Figs 6.29, 6.30, 8.5–8.8)
Professor P. Cole, London (Fig. 10.25)
Dr A. Colville, Nottingham (Figs 1.5, 1.7, 1.8, 4.22, 4.28, 4.33, 6.6, 7.16, 11.20, 11.21, 11.32, 11.33)
Dr M. Franco, Botucatu, Brazil (Figs 8.12, 8.13)
Dr W. Irving, (Figs 1.21–1.23, 1.27–1.29, 6.31–6.33)
Dr I. Johnston, Nottingham (Fig. 7.15)
Professor J. S. P. Jones, Nottingham (Fig. 9.14)
Dr M. Lubani, Farwania, Kuwait (Fig. 8.1)
Dr A. Manhire, Nottingham (Fig. 2.12)
Dr R. Miller, London (Figs 6.4, 6.5, 6.26, 6.36)
Mr W. E. Morgan (Figs 2.14–2.16, 10.5)
Professor M. Razaque, Imphal, India (Fig. 8.18)
Dr D. Ryrie, Nottingham (Fig. 1.15)
Mr F. Salama, Nottingham (Figs 9.5, 9.6)
Dr W. Schell, Durham, USA (Figs 6.25, 8.3, 8.10)
Mr A. Shelton, Nottingham (Fig. 6.11)
Mrs C. Stacey, Nottingham (Figs 10.14, 10.15)
Dr H. Tubbs, Stoke-on-Trent (Figs 12.1, 12.2)
Dr M. Wilkinson, Nottingham (Figs 10.26, 10.27)

We are particularly indebted for help and co-operation from the Departments of Radiology and Histopathology, City Hospital, Nottingham and the Public Health Laboratory Service, Nottingham, Mrs Sue Hurst of the Photographic and Illustration Department, City Hospital, Nottingham and the guidance and patience of Annalisa Page and Simon Armstrong of the Editorial Staff of Chapman and Hall. Professor Tom Marrie kindly took on the task of writing the foreword for our book and for this we are extremely grateful to him.

Foreword

Pneumonia is one of the most difficult problems that I encounter as an infectious disease consultant. Our overall mortality rate for community-acquired pneumonia is 20%, and an etiological diagnosis is made in only about half of our patients. While a small number of microbial agents account for many pneumonia cases there are well over 50 etiological agents that are not uncommon causes. The clinical manifestations of pneumonia vary considerably, from a very mild illness to that of a rapidly progressive, overwhelming infection such as pneumococcal pneumonia in the asplenic host. Likewise, fulminant *Legionella* pneumonia can result in death in an otherwise healthy individual within 24 hours.

The last two decades have seen remarkable changes in the field of pneumonia – new pathogens have been identified – *Legionella pneumophila* and multiple other *Legionella* species, *Chlamydia pneumoniae*; and marked changes in the population at risk for pneumonia. The elderly are the largest growing segment of the population in the UK and in North America. As a result nursing-home acquired pneumonia, with its own set of difficulties in diagnosis and therapy, now accounts for 10–15% of all cases of pneumonia requiring admission to hospital. AIDS has made *Pneumocystis carinii*, *Cryptococcus neoformans* and multiresistant *M. tuberculosis* common problems with which all physicians must be familiar. The success of our transplantation programs has led to a large number of renal, cardiac and bone marrow transplant patients in the community and in our hospitals. These immunocompromized patients must have an etiological diagnosis made when they develop pneumonia so that appropriate therapy can be initiated. Invasive techniques including open lung biopsy are often necessary to make such a diagnosis. The multifaceted clinical problem of pneumonia demands an in-depth, up-to-date knowledge base on the part of the physician. In order to treat pneumonia successfully one must bring to the problem a logical approach to diagnosis and therapy.

This *Colour Atlas of Respiratory Infections* is an important aid for all those who deal with pneumonia. The atlas is organized into twelve sections, covering the entire spectrum of pneumonia including laboratory diagnosis. The illustration of this particular subject is provided by an excellent selection of chest radiographs demonstrating the wide variation in radiographic manifestations of pneumonia due to many different etiological agents. Special radiographic examinations, such as computed tomography, amplify features visualized on plain radiographs. The gross pathological findings are shown for a number of cases, as are the histological manifestations. It is evident that the authors have used carefully selected material from collections built up over many years. The blend of chest physician, infectious disease physician/microbiologist and pathologist has resulted in a balanced presentation of the clinical, microbiological and pathological features.

This atlas allows for a rapid overview of a complex field. It will especially benefit trainees in infectious diseases, microbiology and respiratory medicine. However, this book should also be part of the library of the general medicine consultant and be readily available to nursing, physiotherapy and medical students – for the latter group it represents a worthwhile investment and they should purchase it.

T. J. Marrie
Division of Infectious Diseases, Victoria General Hospital, Nova Scotia

1. Laboratory diagnosis of respiratory tract infection

INTRODUCTION

The laboratory diagnosis of respiratory tract infections (RTI) draws on a range of tests of varying complexity, sensitivity and specificity. Gram stain and culture continue as the mainstay of diagnosis for most common bacterial infections. Specific infections may require special media for isolation, as in the case of *Mycoplasma pneumoniae* and *Legionella pneumophila* infections. If mycobacterial infection is suspected, examination of sputum for acid- and alcohol-fast or auramine-fluorescing bacilli is indicated. Virus identification can be rapid with the use of specific antibody-labelled reagents but is generally slower when virus isolation or evidence of seroconversion is sought.

The value of sputum bacteriology is a frequent source of debate, since it is very much dependent on the quality of the sample. Difficulties with expectoration, previous antibiotic exposure, contamination by normal oropharyngeal flora and delays in transportation all affect the ability of the laboratory to establish a microbiological diagnosis. Equally important is the range of tests set up against a particular specimen owing to the variety of pathogens responsible for RTI. Apart from conventional cultural techniques, other methods include the use of specific stains such as fluorescein-labelled antibodies against agents such as influenza and respiratory syncytial virus; these may be used on nasopharyngeal secretions, expectorated sputum or lavage material obtained at bronchoscopy according to the nature of the infection under investigation. It is important to stress the need for accurate clinical details to accompany any request for microbiological investigation since this determines the choice and conduct of the laboratory tests. Blood cultures, when positive, are extremely helpful and provide a specific diagnosis. Unfortunately bacteraemia is an uncommon accompaniment of RTI apart from community-acquired pneumococcal pneumonia, where about 10–20% of untreated patients will have positive blood cultures.

Other non-cultural techniques for microbial identification include antigen detection using various systems such as countercurrent immunoelectrophoresis and latex agglutination. Examination of samples other than sputum may also be helpful and these include serum, urine and pleural aspirates. The latter should also be submitted for conventional Gram stain and culture examination.

A retrospective diagnosis of infection can be made by seeking a specific antibody response in paired serum samples to a particular pathogen. Conventionally a battery of microbial antigens is tested which includes a variety of common viral and bacterial pathogens. However, if a specific disease is clinically suspected this should be stated, since the laboratory will either set up or forward samples to a reference centre to test for the particular infecting organism. The complexity of serological diagnosis is exemplified by *Legionella* infections where many different species and serogroups of specific species have been associated with human disease. However, *Legionella pneumophila*, serogroup 1, remains the commonest pathogen and is usually screened for. Many of these laboratory aspects of diagnosis are illustrated.

SPUTUM MICROSCOPY

Sputum provides one of the most important clinical samples for the laboratory diagnosis of lower RTI. Unfortunately patients are often poorly instructed in its collection, which is often made the responsibility of inexperienced nursing staff. This inevitably leads to poor quality specimens which fail to produce meaningful information. Only about two thirds of patients during the acute phase of a bacterial pneumonia will be able to produce a satisfactory sputum specimen spontaneously. The others in their attempts to provide a specimen will produce saliva or no sample at all. Any 'sputum' that is produced will inevitably be contaminated by oropharyngeal material and organisms, sometimes making the interpretation of Gram stain and culture difficult. It is the responsibility of the clinician, the physiotherapist (Fig. 1.1) or the nurse to send the best possible specimen to the laboratory. A useful guide to the

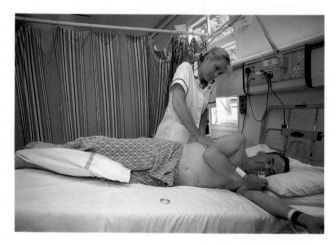

Fig. 1.1 A physiotherapist can be helpful in aiding a patient with bronchial secretions to produce a good sputum.

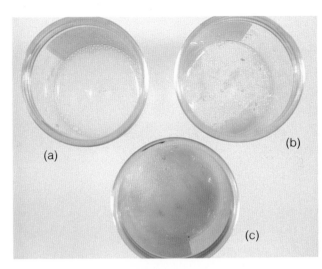

Fig. 1.2 Examples of different sputa. (a) Salivary sample of little value. **(b)** Mucopurulent. **(c)** Purulent.

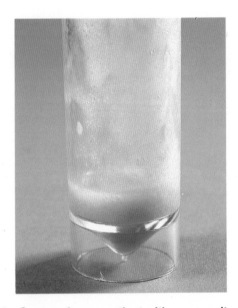

Fig. 1.3 Sputum from a patient with community-acquired *Klebsiella pneumoniae* pneumonia showing a purulent, blood-stained appearance.

bronchial ulceration from a neoplasm but may also point to an infected pulmonary infarct or bleeding into an aspergilloma. Altered blood renders the sputum 'rusty' in appearance and typifies the early stage of pneumococcal pneumonia. Three types of 'sputum' specimens are illustrated (Fig. 1.2). Sometime the macroscopic appearance of the sputum is said to give an indication of the likely pathogen (Fig. 1.3). On occasions, a physiotherapist can be extremely helpful in obtaining a deep cough specimen of sputum (Fig. 1.1) although in a seriously ill or toxic patient with pneumonia the likely benefits from obtaining such a sample must be weighed against the stress caused and should not delay the commencement of appropriate antibiotic therapy.

Sputum induction using 3% normal saline delivered by ultrasonic nebulizer is an inexpensive, non-invasive and helpful technique for obtaining bronchoalveolar secretions. In experienced hands it is particularly useful for diagnosing pneumocystis pneumonia in AIDS or other immunocompromised patients (Fig. 1.4). Microscopic examination is also important in differentiating expectorated sputum from upper airways secretions. The latter (Fig. 1.5) shows a predominance of epithelial cells and on Gram stain a variety of microorganisms typical of the normal oropharyngeal bacterial flora. This contrasts with the appearance of a good quality sputum sample from a patient with pneumococcal pneumo-

quality of a specimen can be obtained by its macroscopic appearance.

Macroscopic examination of an expectorated sputum sample is often sufficient to indicate whether it is primarily sputum or entirely or predominantly saliva. Sputum is customarily described macroscopically as mucoid, mucopurulent or purulent, whilst the presence of frank or altered blood provides additional valuable information. Purulent sputum mixed with bright red blood may indicate

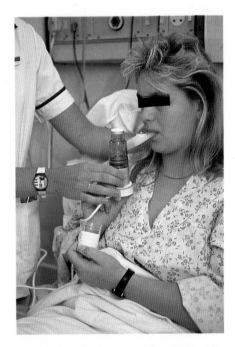

Fig. 1.4 Nebulized hypertonic saline by an ultrasonic nebulizer can be a useful method of sputum induction.

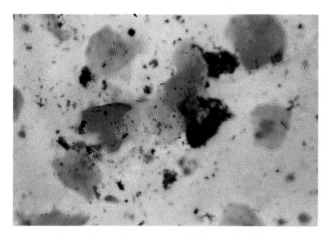

Fig. 1.5 Gram stain of a poor sputum specimen showing numerous epithelial cells and a variety of bacteria present in the normal oropharynx.

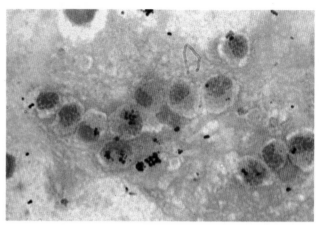

Fig. 1.7 Gram stain of sputum from a patient with staphylococcal pneumonia showing many pus cells and Gram-positive cocci, some of which are intracellular.

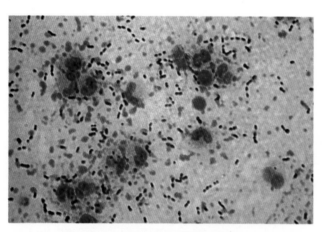

Fig. 1.6 Sputum from a patient with pneumococcal **pneumonia.** Note presence of pus cells and large numbers of Gram-positive diplococci, some in short chains. A clear zone is visible around some of them and represents abundant capsular material.

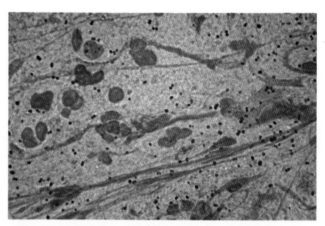

Fig. 1.8 Gram stain of sputum from a patient with an **infective exacerbation of chronic bronchitis.** This shows numerous Gram-negative diplococci typical of *Moraxella (Branhamella)* catarrhalis.

nia (Fig. 1.6) where the Gram stain provides valuable information on the presence of pus cells, and the typical staining appearance of pneumococci. *Staphylococcus aureus* pneumonia, although relatively uncommon, is a most serious and virulent infection that may occur de novo or as a complication of influenza. Early information to direct antibiotic choice may be gained by examining the sputum for the presence of typical Gram-positive cocci in clusters (Fig. 1.7), seen both intracellularly and extracellularly. This appearance provides a presumptive microbiological diagnosis and is an indication for parental anti-staphylococcal therapy.

Sputum examination is less widely requested in

patients with chronic bronchitis where infective exacerbations have largely been associated with *Haemophilus influenzae* infection. However, the increasing association of *Moraxella (Branhamella) catarrhalis* with infective exacerbations and the increasing resistance of *H. influenzae* to ampicillin suggests that more regular examination of the purulent specimens from these patients may be appropriate. Figure 1.8 shows a Gram-stained sputum sample with numerous pus cells and Gram-negative diplococci typical of *M. catarrhalis*. The significance of this organism lies in its frequent resistance to ampicillin and related drugs as a result of beta-lactamase production.

Patients with infective exacerbations of chronic

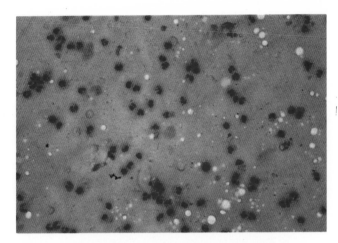

Fig. 1.9 Gram stain of sputum from a patient with bacterial pneumonia revealing many pus cells but no organisms; due to prior antibiotics.

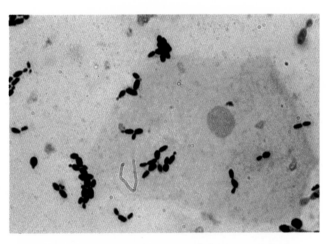

Fig. 1.10 An example of an unsatisfactory sputum sample. Note the presence of epithelial cells and yeasts compatible with contamination by oropharyngeal secretions. The patient had received antibiotics before admission to hospital.

airways disease may require admission to hospital. They will have frequently received antibiotics in the community and the effect this has on sputum microbiology is demonstrated in Fig. 1.9. No organisms are visible despite the presence of large numbers of pus cells. A similar effect may be seen in community-acquired pneumococcal pneumonia where bacteria rapidly disappear from the sputum after antibiotic exposure. Broad-spectrum antibiotics also encourage the overgrowth of Gram-negative bacilli and yeasts and Fig. 1.10 shows a poor quality sputum sample containing epithelial cells with overgrowth of yeasts; such an appearance may or may not be associated with clinical evidence of oral candidiasis.

SPUTUM CULTURE

Sputum is generally cultured on blood agar, which is a general purpose medium that supports the growth of many common respiratory bacterial pathogens. However, *H. influenzae* grows best on chocolate blood agar in which the blood has been preheated.

Figure 1.11 illustrates the typical growth and sensitivity pattern of *Streptococcus pneumoniae* on blood agar; the dark green (alpha-haemolysis) reflects the area of growth and is clearly distinguished from the clear unaltered zone surrounding the paper disk. These disks contain bile salts (OP), to which the pneumococcus is exquisitely sensitive, and bacitracin (BA) which differentiates pneumococci from other oral viridans streptococci. The remaining disks indicate the sensitivity of the pneumococcus to penicillin (PG), methicillin (MT) (and by inference flucloxacillin) and ampicillin (AP).

By way of contrast, Fig. 1.12 shows the appearance of *Klebsiella pneumoniae*, which is an occasional but serious cause of pneumonia, particularly among hospitalized patients and those with underlying disorders such as alchoholism. The antibiotic sensitivity profile of this organism growing in the two outer zones compared with a control organism in the centre zone shows sensitivity to ciprofloxacin (bottom right), cefotaxime (bottom left) and gentamicin (top left), but resistance to ampicillin (top right) as a result of beta-lactamase production.

The importance of careful sample collection and selection by microscopy is illustrated in Fig. 1.13, where a poorly collected sputum specimen on culture has yielded a range of respiratory bacteria of

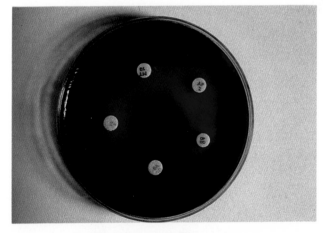

Fig. 1.11 Characteristic sensitivity pattern of *Streptococcus pneumoniae*. Note zones of inhibition around discs containing ampicillin (AP), methicillin (MT) and optochin (bile salt) and absent zone around bacitracin (BA).

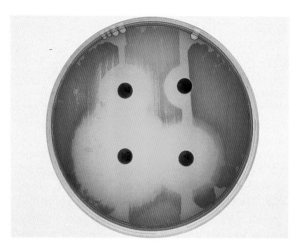

**Fig. 1.12   Sensitivity pattern of *Klebsiella pneumoniae*
(outer sections) compared with a fully sensitive control
strain (central section).** The zones of inhibition are
equivalent for ciprofloxacin (bottom right), cefotaxime
(bottom left) and gentamicin (top left) but demonstrate
resistance to ampicillin (top right) where no zone is visible.
Klebsiella pneumoniae is resistant to ampicillin by virtue of
beta-lactamase production.   ·

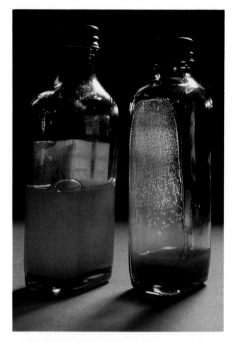

**Fig. 1.14   Positive blood culture from a patient with
Staphylococcus aureus pneumonia.** Note turbid broth in
left-hand bottle and numerous colonies on agar slant in
right-hand bottle.

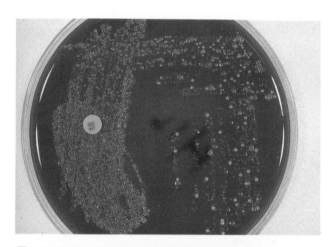

**Fig. 1.13   Blood agar plate showing growth of
numerous respiratory commensals from a poor quality
sputum specimen contaminated by oropharyngeal
secretions.**

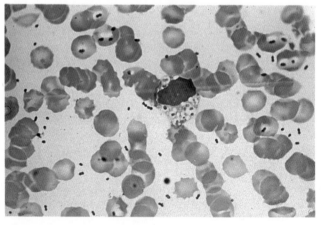

**Fig. 1.15   Blood film of patient with overwhelming
pneumococcal septicaemia.** Note enormous numbers of
Gram-positive diplococci. The patient had previously
undergone splenectomy.

varying colonial morphology. There is no zone
around the bile salt (OP) disk, thus confirming the
absence of the pneumococcus.

BLOOD CULTURES

One to two sets of blood cultures should be collected
from hospitalized patients with pneumonia regard-
less of whether the infection arises in the community
or hospital. Although only 10–20% of patients will
be bacteraemic, a positive result provides valuable
information on the nature of the infection and its
severity. Figure 1.14 illustrates a typical two-bottle
blood culture system containing broth with turbid
growth (left) and an integral agar slope on which
bacterial colonies are growing (right). Pneumococcal
pneumonia is the commonest infection to be associ-

ated with bacteraemia which occurs with varying frequency according to pneumococcal serotype; more virulent serotypes such as serotype 3 are more likely to produce bacteraemic infection. In patients who are hyposplenic (e.g. sickle cell disease) or asplenic (e.g. congenital or surgical removal), pneumococcal bacteraemia may be fulminant as illustrated in Fig. 1.15, where the number of bacteria present is so great that they are visible in the blood film. The patient had had a splenectomy some years earlier following a road traffic accident.

NON-CULTURAL DIAGNOSTIC METHODS

Countercurrent immunoelectrophoresis and latex agglutination

One of the difficulties inherent in the microbiological confirmation of respiratory tract infections is the occasional insensitivity of cultural methods and necessity for a good quality sputum specimen. Alternative methods of diagnosis have been aimed at detecting surface antigenic structures with the use of specific high titre antibody preparations. At present these investigations are not universally available in diagnostic laboratories but they do provide valuable early information on the possible microbiological diagnosis.

The diagnosis of bacterial infections by antigen detection in expectorated sputum, infected pleural fluid, serum or urine has proved most helpful when diagnosing pneumococcal infections. The diagnostic specificity of concentrated urine, serum and pleural fluid assay is very high and the sensitivity is greater than for cultural methods. For sputum assay, the sensitivity in reported studies is 68–94% and there is increasing evidence of good specificity for diagnosing pneumococcal pneumonia.

Most experience has been gained by using the techniques of countercurrent immunoelectrophoresis (CIEP) and latex agglutination, which both use a high titre polyvalent pneumococcal antiserum (Omniserum), available through the Statens Serum Institute, Copenhagen. The apparatus for CIEP is illustrated in Fig. 1.16 and consists of a power pack and electrophoretic tank which contains buffer connected to a glass slide, on which is a solidified buffered agar layer, by a filter paper wick through which the current passes. The agar plate has two wells of approximately one millimetre diameter, separated by 0.5 cm. The test sample is placed in the cathodal well while the antibody fills the anodal well (Fig. 1.17). On passing a current for approximately 30 minutes the presence of negatively charged

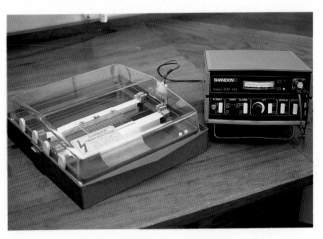

Fig. 1.16 Typical equipment required for countercurrent immunoelectrophoresis (CIEP) for detection of pneumococcal antigen.

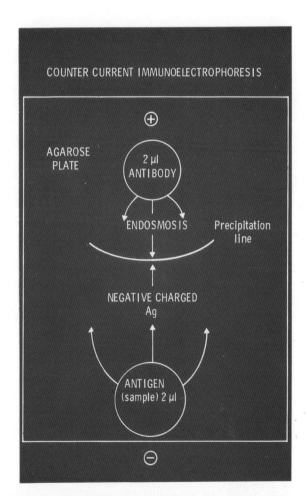

Fig. 1.17 Schematic arrangement of countercurrent immunoelectrophoresis (CIEP) for antigen detection. Antibody (e.g. pneumococcal) is placed in the anodal well and the test sample (antigen) in the cathodal well. In the presence of an electrical field antigen and antibody meet to produce a precipitin line of identification.

pneumococcal polysaccharide antigen will be recognized by the formation of a precipitin line between the two wells.

The system allows multiple samples to be tested simultaneously, together with positive and negative controls (Fig. 1.18). CIEP has proved extremely valuable in our hands in the diagnosis of pneumococcal infection, especially in the absence of positive cultures. Most pneumococcal serotypes can be identified by this technique but occasional serotypes (e.g. serotype 14) may not be detected unless the buffer pH is adjusted.

An alternative system for the diagnosis of pneumococcal disease uses latex agglutination (Fig. 1.19). Latex particles are coated with polyvalent

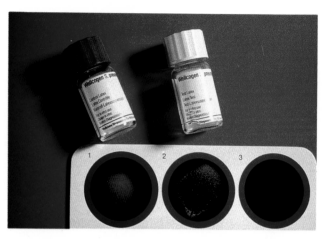

Fig. 1.20 Pneumococcal antigen detection by latex agglutination. A positive reaction is visible in the centre well. A control well is on the left.

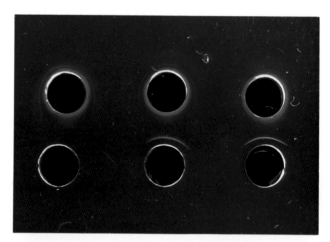

Fig. 1.18 Precipitation lines formed in agarose plate denote presence of pneumococcal antigen in test specimen, by CIEP. Control pair of wells on left.

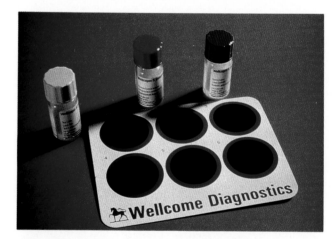

Fig. 1.19 Commercial kit for detection of pneumococcal polysaccharide antigen by latex agglutination. Test sample and reagent are mixed and gently rocked on a glass slide until agglutination occurs.

pneumococcal antiserum and when gently mixed with a broth suspension of *Strep. pneumoniae* produce agglutination of the latex particles, which become visible. This is illustrated in Fig. 1.20. Although not intended for direct testing of body fluids, published experience suggests that latex agglutination can be valuable when testing sputum direct, and has a degree of sensitivity that is slightly better than CIEP. However, this must be balanced against local experience in the availability and use of either technique. The ability to diagnose other bacterial pneumonias by these or other antigen-detecting techniques has been disappointing owing to the limited availability of suitable high titre antiserum. There are some favourable reports on the diagnosis of *H. influenzae* infection in children where type *b* strains are more prevalent and for which a suitable antiserum exists.

Fluorescent antibody systems

Other methods used in the acute diagnosis of respiratory infection include the use of fluorescein-labelled antibody systems for the diagnosis of RSV (respiratory syncytial virus) and influenza virus infections and more recently *Legionella pneumophila* and *Pneumocystis carinii* infections; the latter uses a monoclonal antibody. Figure 1.21 illustrates a positive direct immunofluorescent stain for RSV in a tracheal aspirate, while Fig. 1.22 demonstrates positive fluorescence for influenza A in nasopharyngeal material. Fluorescent antibody systems are also used as confirmatory tests during virus isolation in tissue culture. Fig. 1.23 shows positive immunofluorescence for RSV in tissue culture.

The range of such rapid diagnostic tests is still

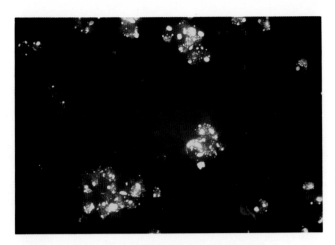

Fig. 1.21   Direct immunofluorescent antibody demonstration of RSV (respiratory syncytial virus) in a tracheal aspirate.

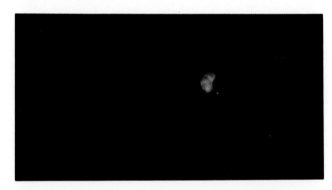

Fig. 1.22   Influenza A in nasopharyngeal aspirate demonstrated by direct fluorescent antibody staining. ×400.

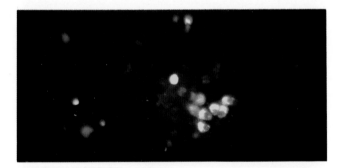

Fig. 1.23   Nasopharyngeal secretions from a child with acute bronchiolitis stained with fluorescein-labelled anti-RSV (respiratory syncytial virus) antibody. Both positive and negative fluorescing cells are visible.

limited although progress with DNA probes and techniques such as the polymerase chain reaction (PCR) are encouraging. In the case of virus infections much emphasis is still placed on tissue culture using various cell lines.

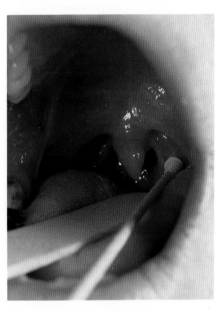

Fig. 1.24   To obtain an effective throat swab specimen, the stick swab must be rubbed vigorously on the tonsillar pillars or the posterior pharyngeal wall and not on the tongue or buccal mucosa.

Samples suitable for culture other than sputum include throat swabs and nasopharyngeal aspirates. A throat swab is obtained by vigorous brushing of the posterior pharyngeal wall and the tonsillar bed; the infected epithelial cells obtained should be transported to the laboratory in viral transport medium (Fig. 1.24). A nasopharyngeal aspirate is obtained by passing a fine cannula pernasally to the nasopharyngeal space, which is then irrigated with millilitres of saline (Fig. 1.25).

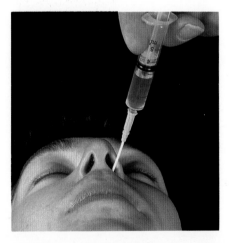

Fig. 1.25   Nasopharyngeal aspirate. A fine catheter has been passed pernasally into the nasopharyngeal space and a few millilitres of saline instilled and sucked back. Such specimens can be suitable for both viral culture and direct immunofluorescent staining for viruses.

These samples are inoculated on to a suitable cell line and following several days incubation result in characteristic morphological changes known as a cytopathic effect (CPE). For example, Fig. 1.26 illustrates a normal HEp2 cell line composed of small uniform cuneiform cells. Following inoculation with respiratory secretions from a patient with adenovirus infection a typical CPE effect is observed (Fig. 1.27).

Figure 1.28 illustrates the typical syncytial appearance produced by RSV-infected HEp2 cells.

Alternative tissue culture systems make use of the alteration of surface epitopes in virus-infected cells. Under some circumstances this allows absorption of red blood cells which then act as an indicator of virus-infected cells. Figure 1.29 shows the typical appearance of haemadsorption of monkey kidney cells infected with influenza A virus.

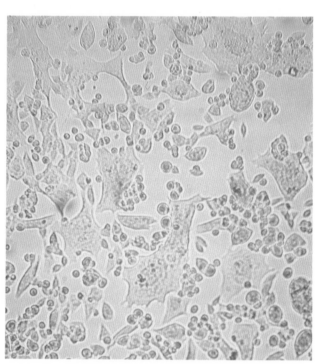

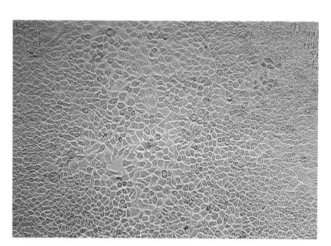

Fig. 1.26   Normal appearance of an HEp2 (human epithelial tumour cell line) tissue culture monolayer used for virus isolation.

Fig. 1.28   Tissue culture of HEp2 cells showing typical syncytial formation caused by respiratory syncytial virus.

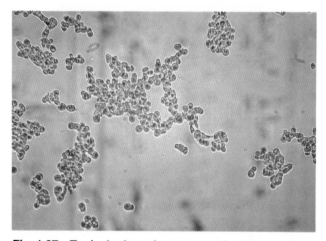

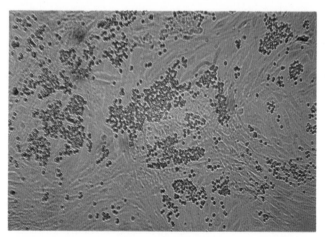

Fig. 1.27   Typical adenovirus cytopathic effect in HEp2 cells.

Fig. 1.29   Positive haemadsorption test in a monkey kidney cell infected with influenza A virus.

Serodiagnosis

A further method widely used in the diagnosis of respiratory infections is the demonstration of type-specific antibody responses which develop in response to infection. By collecting baseline and convalescent serum at approximately 7–10 days,

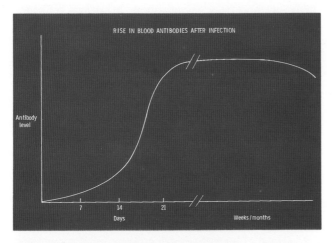

Fig. 1.30 Diagrammatic demonstration of antibody response against time following infection.

although in the case of *Legionella pneumophila* infection a sample at six weeks may be necessary, a variety of test systems can be employed to detect this seroconversion (Fig. 1.30). One of the most widely used systems is based on complement fixation. In the presence of type-specific antibody, complement becomes fixed and therefore unavailable for red blood lysis when such cells are added as an indicator of positivity. For example, Fig. 1.31 demonstrates seroconversion to influenza B virus infection in the convalescent sample where a titre of > 160 has resulted compared with the acute sample. Other infections tested for in this battery of complement fixation tests include influenza A, parainfluenza, RSV adenovirus, psittacosis/lymphogranuloma venereum (which use a common antigen), Q fever and *Mycoplasma pneumoniae*. Figure 1.32 illustrates seroconversion to psittacosis, again to a titre of > 160, in the convalescent sample. Such test systems by their nature provide retrospective information on a particular infection and are therefore more valuable in providing epidemiological information on the prevalence of infections.

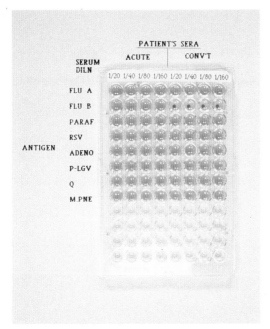

Fig. 1.31 Respiratory serology (1). Paired serum samples demonstrating seroconversion to influenza B with a titre of 160 in the convalescent sample. Complement fixation is indicated by the clumping of the added red blood cells.

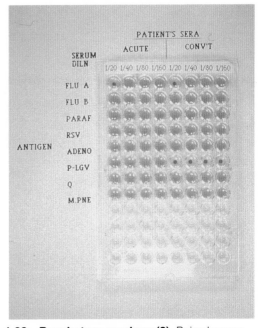

Fig. 1.32 Respiratory serology (2). Paired serum samples demonstrating seroconversion to the psittacosislymphogranuloma venereum (P-LGV) antigen used to detect recent chlamydial infection. The convalescent serum shows a titre of 160. The titre to influenza A has remained unchanged at 20 which is consistent with past infection. Complement fixation is indicated by the clumping of added red blood cells.

OTHER SAMPLES

In addition to microbiological tests, other laboratory investigations should be considered. Hypoalbuminaemia is not uncommon with severe pneumonia related to the toxaemia and the hypercatabolic state that accompanies any serious infection. Hypoatraemia is not uncommon and not only reflects fluid and electrolyte depletion but may indicate inappropriate ADH secretion which accompanies either the pneumonia or reflects hormone secretions from an underlying bronchogenic neoplasm. Liver enzyme abnormalities are also common and relate to severe infection although haemolysis may contribute to the raised bilirubin seen in some patients, particularly with *Mycoplasma pneumoniae* infection. A high white cell count is a feature of bacterial infections whereas those with atypical pneumonia tend to have a normal or only slightly raised white cell count.

FURTHER READING

Bartlett, J. G., Ryan, K. J., Smith, T. F. and Wilson, W. R. (1987) *Cumitech 7A: Laboratory diagnosis of lower respiratory trace infections* (Co-ordinating editor J. A. Washington II), pp. 1–18. American Society for Microbiology, Washington, DC.

Fung, J. C. and Tilton, R. C. (1985) Detection of bacterial antigens by counter-immunoelectrophoresis, coagglutination, and latex agglutination. In *Manual of Clinical Microbiology*, 4th edn (eds E. H. Lennette, A. Balows, W. J. Hausler Jr and H. J. Shadomy), pp. 883–90, American Society of Microbiology, Washington DC.

Leland, D. S. and French, M. L. V. (1988) Virus isolation and identification. In *Laboratory Diagnosis of Infectious Diseases, Principles and Practice*, Vol. II, *Viral, Rickettsial and Chlamydial Disease* (eds E. H. Lennette, P. Halonen and F. A. Murphy), Chapter 3. Springer-Verlag, New York.

Spencer, R. C. and Philp, J. R. (1973) Effect of previous antimicrobial therapy on bacteriological findings in patients with primary pneumonia. *Lancet*, **ii**, 349–51.

Woodhead, M. A., Macfarlane, J. T., Finch, R. G. and McCracken, J. S. (1990) A comparison of countercurrent immunoelectrophoresis and latex agglutination for the detection of pneumococcal antigen in a community-based pneumonia study. *Serodiagnosis and Immunotherapy in Infectious Disease*, **4**, 159–65.

2. *Invasive Techniques for the Investigation of Respiratory Tract Infections*

INTRODUCTION

There are a number of invasive techniques available which can be useful in identifying the likely pathogen causing a respiratory infection (Table 2.1). The strategy adopted to investigate an individual patient will be based on several factors, including the severity of the infection, the investigational and laboratory resources available, the sensitivity, specificity and risk of the procedure and the likely spectrum of pathogens in a particular clinical situation. At one extreme there will be the previously fit adult who presents to his general practitioner with a mild community-acquired lower respiratory infection, shows a rapid response to therapy and requires no investigation. At the other end of the spectrum is the patient treated with immunosuppressive therapy who develops fever and progressive lung shadowing, and in whom the spectrum of potential pathogens is wide and the necessity for making an accurate diagnosis urgent. In such a patient, early invasive investigations may be the most efficient approach for identifying a pathogen and planning appropriate therapy. Invasive techniques performed on an individual in extremis and already on broad-spectrum antibacterial, antifungal and antiviral therapy rarely yield helpful results.

This chapter deals with the practical aspects of obtaining speciment.

TRANSTRACHEAL SALINE INJECTION

This is a useful, quick and successful method of obtaining a deep cough specimen of sputum. The

---

Table 2.1   List of available techniques that are used for investigating lower respiratory tract infections

Transtracheal saline injection
Transtracheal aspiration
Fibreoptic bronchoscopy with:
  Bronchial aspirates
  Bronchial lavage
  Bronchial biopsies
  Bronchoalveolar lavage
  Protected specimen brush
  Transbronchial lung biopsies
Percutaneous fine needle aspirates
Open lung biopsy
Pleural fluid aspirate
Pleural biopsy

---

brisk injection of 5 ml of saline into the trachea, via a 21 gauge needle inserted through the cricothyroid membrane, will usually stimulate the production of a deep cough specimen of sputum and obviate the need for more invasive techniques (Fig. 2.1).

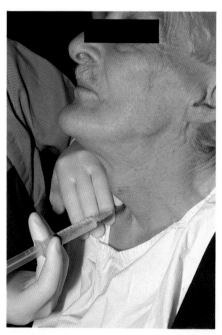

Fig. 2.1   A transtracheal injection of saline usually stimulates a deep cough specimen of lower respiratory secretions.

TRANSTRACHEAL ASPIRATION

In this technique, a sterile narrow 14 gauge catheter is fed through a needle introduced into the trachea,

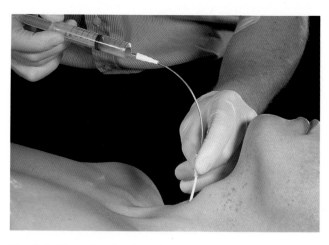

Fig. 2.2   Transtracheal aspiration is performed by passing a catheter through the cricothyroid membrane.

via the cricothyroid membrane, under local anaesthesia and is advanced towards the carina. Two millilitres of normal saline can then be instilled and a specimen obtained by firm negative pressure on the syringe as the catheter is withdrawn. Low patient acceptability, local bleeding and traumatic surgical emphysema have now made this technique much less popular than bronchoscopic methods (Fig. 2.2).

BRONCHOSCOPIC METHODS

Fibreoptic bronchoscopy is a widely available and safe technique that allows access to the lower respiratory tract for obtaining samples, including:

1. Bronchial aspirates.
2. Bronchial lavage.
3. Bronchoalveolar lavage.
4. Transbronchial lung biopsies.
5. Protected specimen brush samples.

Fibreoptic bronchoscopy is normally performed under local anaesthesia with or without sedation. The technique is suitable for use in the endoscopy unit, on the ward, in the intensive care unit and in the operating theatre (Fig. 2.3).

Bronchial aspirates and bronchial lavage

Bronchial aspirates and bronchial lavage using small quantities of saline can provide useful specimens from patients with simple community bacterial infections but can produce misleading results from patients with nosocomial infections or receiving assisted ventilation where bacterial colonization of the airways is not uncommon.

Bronchoalveolar lavage

The technique of bronchoalveolar lavage varies. Usually the bronchoscope is wedged into a segmental bronchus and aliquots of normal saline at body temperature are instilled into the segment until a volume of at least 30 ml of effluent can be collected by suction. The chest radiograph in Fig. 2.4 illustrates the bronchoscope introduced into the right middle lobe bronchus followed by instillation of only 15 ml of a radiopaque lavage solution. Note the extensive alveolar filling even with this small volume. Generally, 100–150 ml of saline are required. The technique is very safe but a fall in arterial oxygen tension is common and patients should receive oxygen therapy during and after the procedure.

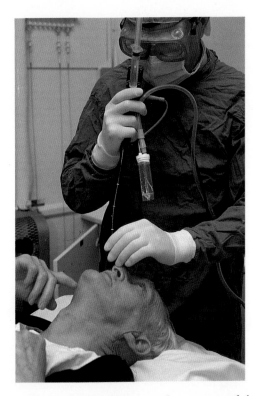

Fig. 2.3 Fibreoptic bronchoscopy is a very useful technique for obtaining lower respiratory secretions.

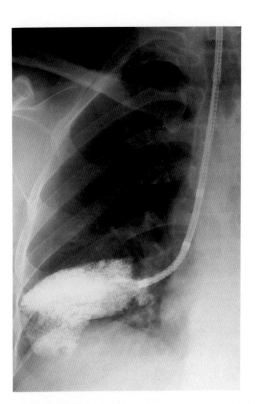

Fig. 2.4 Limited bronchoalveolar lavage of right middle lobe using radiopaque solution.

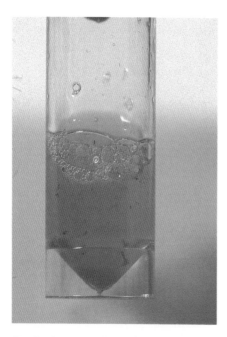

Fig. 2.5 Typical material from bronchoalveolar lavage from a patient with bacterial pneumonia.

A typical example of aspirated material following bronchoalveolar lavage in a patient found to have bacterial pneumonia is shown in Fig. 2.5.

Protected specimen brush

The protected specimen brush (PSB) is used to obtain the sample from the bronchiolar level uncontaminated either by the bronchoscopic channel or during passage through the major bronchi. The extended PSB can be seen protruding from the end of the bronchoscope in Fig. 2.6. A protective gelatine plug occludes the end of the outer plastic cover until the inner protective yellow plastic cannula is extended when the PSB is in position within a segmental bronchus.

The chest radiograph in Fig. 2.7 shows the PSB (arrow) protruding several inches from the end of the bronchoscope to obtain samples deep in the right middle lobe.

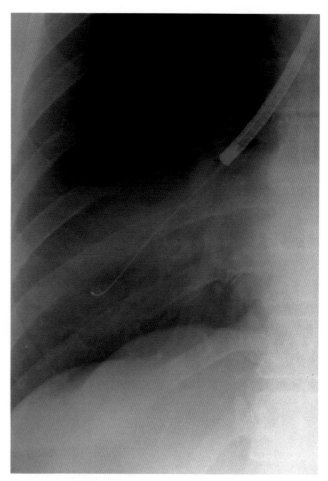

Fig. 2.7 Chest radiograph of protected specimen brush in right middle lobe.

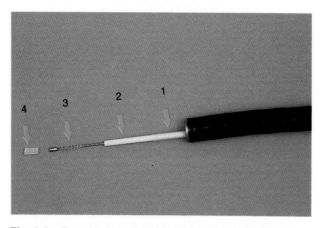

Fig. 2.6 Extended protected specimen brush. Note the outer plastic cover (arrow 1), and the inner protective yellow plastic cover (arrow 2) with the microbiological brush pushed out (arrow 3). The protective gelatin plug occludes the end of the outer cover (arrow 4) until specimens are obtained.

Transbronchial lung biopsy

Small specimens of lung tissue can be obtained for microbiological and histological examination with a transbronchial lung biopsy performed through the fibreoptic bronchoscope. Figure 2.8 illustrates the open forceps (arrow), which can be seen deep in the

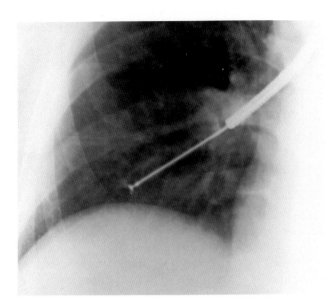

Fig. 2.8 Chest radiograph of transbronchial lung biopsy being performed.

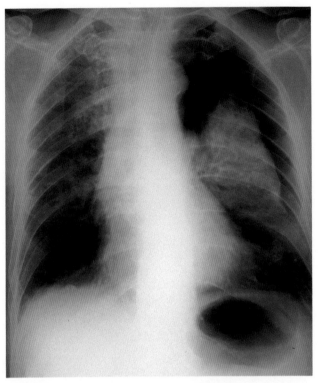

Fig. 2.10 Chest radiograph showing a left pneumothorax following transbronchial lung biopsy.

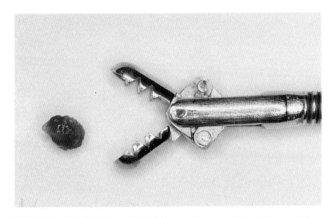

Fig. 2.9 Typical toothed biopsy forceps together with a good transbronchial biopsy of consolidated lung.

right lower lobe during a biopsy being performed under radiographic screening.

A close-up view shows the typical toothed biopsy forceps together with a transbronchial biopsy of consolidated lung. Normally several biopsies are taken from different segments of one lung (Fig. 2.9).

Complications of transbronchial biopsy include haemorrhage and pneumothorax. Because of this, biopsies should not be taken from both lungs during the procedure or performed on patients receiving positive pressure ventilation, as may occur in an intensive care unit. The chest radiograph in Fig. 2.10 shows a left pneumothorax following a transbronchial biopsy in a patient shown to have *Pneumocystis carinii* pneumonia. Tube drainage was required.

In patients who are thrombocytopenic or have

uncorrectable bleeding problems, transbronchial biopsy should not be performed and broncho-alveolar lavage, which is relatively safe, should be considered instead.

PERCUTANEOUS FINE NEEDLE ASPIRATES

Small samples of lung secretions can be obtained by this method, which can be performed at the bedside. A fine gauge needle (e.g. 25 gauge) is advanced into the lung, sometimes through a short thicker intro-ducer needle which is also used to give local anaesthesia to the chest wall and parietal sub-pleural area. After injecting 1 or 2 ml of saline into the infected lung area, negative pressure is exerted on the syringe to withdraw a sample (Fig. 2.11). The sample is immediately transported in Ringer's lactate solution to the laboratory. Complications are un-usual in experienced hands, with pneumothorax or haemoptysis, requiring intervention, occurring in about 1% of procedures.

On occasions radiographic screening is required for the accurate placement of a fine needle into the infected portion of the lung, prior to aspiration or screw biopsy (Fig. 2.12).

In the case shown in Fig. 2.13 the needle has been

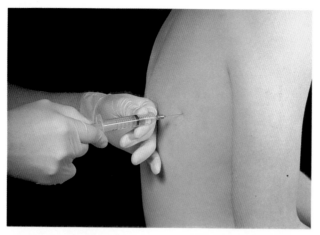

Fig. 2.11 Percutaneous fine needle aspirate is a useful technique for obtaining a sample of 'lung juice' from consolidated areas.

placed under radiographic screening into the consolidated right middle lobe prior to obtaining aspirates for culture.

OPEN LUNG BIOPSY

Open lung biopsy can be very valuable in certain circumstances, including the differentiation of the many causes of infective and non-infective lung shadowing in the immunocompromised individual. It results in a high diagnostic yield although the risks of a general anaesthetic and the procedure have to be weighed against the needs for a definitive diagnosis in seriously ill patients.

The biopsy can be made through a short submammary incision (Fig. 2.14). A tongue of lung tissue is

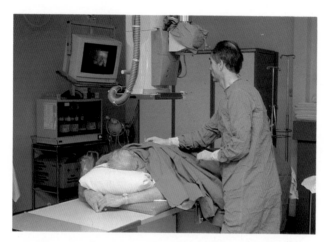

Fig. 2.12 Radiographic screening may be necessary to accurately place a fine needle percutaneously into an area of lung shadowing.

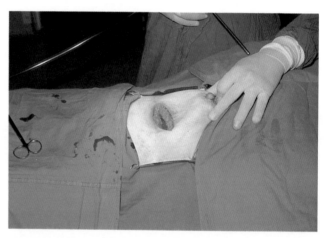

Fig. 2.14 A short submammary incision used for open lung biopsy.

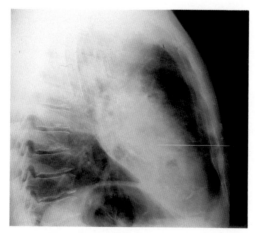

Fig. 2.13 In this case, the needle has been placed into the right middle lobe under radiographic screening.

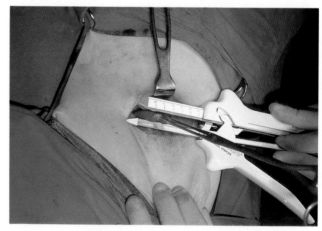

Fig. 2.15 A tongue of lung tissue is removed with the aid of the automatic stapler device. Biopsies from more than one lobe can be obtained.

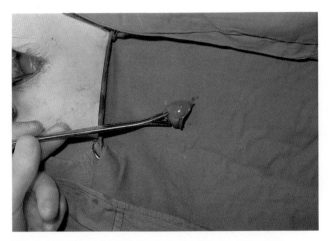

Fig. 2.16 Open lung biopsy produces a generous sample of lung tissue.

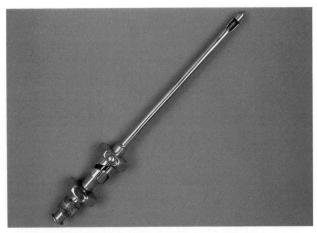

Fig. 2.18 An Abrams pleural biopsy needle. Histological and microbiological examination of pleural biopsies is particularly helpful for making a diagnosis of pleural tuberculosis.

delivered through the incision and a biopsy taken, aided by an automatic stapler device (Fig. 2.15).

The open biopsy produces a generous sample of lung tissue which should be divided in the fresh state so it is suitable for both histological and microbiological examination (Fig. 2.16).

PLEURAL FLUID SAMPLING

Pleural fluid should always be sampled, when detected in the presence of a pneumonia. This allows the exclusion of an empyema and may also identify the cause of the infection.

A diagnostic pleural aspiration can be performed simply at the bedside (Fig. 2.17). Where localization is difficult, it should be performed under ultrasound guidance. For the diagnosis of tuberculous effusions histological examination and culture of pleural biopsies can be particularly helpful. The Abrams biopsy needle is most commonly used (Fig. 2.18). At least one biopsy should always be sent fresh in a few drops of saline to the laboratory for microbiological examination (Fig. 2.19).

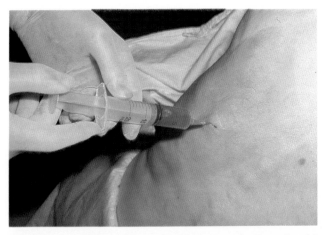

Fig. 2.17 A simple diagnostic pleural aspiration should always be performed if pleural fluid is present in a patient with pneumonia.

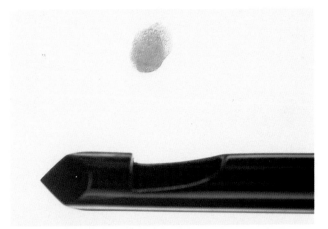

Fig. 2.19 A close-up of the cutting notch of the Abrams needle and a typical pleural biopsy specimen. One sample should always be sent for culture.

FURTHER READING

Bartlett, J. G. (1989) Invasive diagnostic techniques in pulmonary infections. In *Respiratory Infections: Diagnosis and Management*, 2nd edn (ed. J. Pennington), pp. 69–96. Raven Press, New York.

Chastre, J., Fagan, J., Domart, Y. and Gibert, C. (1989) Diagnosis of nosocomial pneumonia in intensive care unit patients. *European Journal of Clinical Microbiology and Infectious Diseases*, **8**, 35–9.

Manresa, F. (1989) Rapid clinical diagnostic methods in respiratory infections. *Current Opinion in Infectious Diseases*, **2**, 536–40.

Manresa, F. and Dorca, J. (1991) Needle aspiration techniques in the diagnosis of pneumonia. *Thorax*, **46**, 601–3.

3. Upper Respiratory Tract Infections

INTRODUCTION

This term includes infections of the sinuses, nasopharynx and larynx. The spectrum of disease varies from the troublesome but trivial common cold through to acute life-threatening stridor from acute epiglottitis.

THE COMMON COLD

This is the most common of acute illnesses with a high infectivity rate. More than 50 different viruses have been implicated. Rhinoviruses are the usual cause although coronaviruses become more important in the winter when respiratory syncytial virus and influenza viruses can also be implicated. On average, people get three colds per year. The incidence is highest in children and decreases with age, particularly if there are no longer children in the household.

Transmission of viruses occurs by droplets produced by coughing or sneezing or direct spread of contaminated secretions on hands or fomites. Shedding of viruses can occur for up to a week in infected individuals. The clinical features of throat discomfort, mild malaise and watery nasal discharge with sneezing are known to everyone. These gradually settle over a few days and complications such as sinusitis are uncommon. Treatment is symptomatic.

SINUSITIS

The maxillary sinuses are usually implicated, probably because of their poor drainage.

The schematic diagram in Fig. 3.1 of the anatomy of the maxillary sinuses shows the inefficient siting of the draining ostium, with much of the sinus being in the lower, dependent position. Even minor swelling of the lining of the ostium can cause blockage and loss of drainage.

Most commonly, sinusitis occurs following an upper respiratory tract infection or allergic rhinitis.

Studies of sinus culture aspirates in community-acquired sinusitis in adults have implicated *Streptococcus pneumoniae* and non-capsulated *Haemophilus influenzae* in the majority of cases. *Moraxella catarrhalis*, anaerobic and aerobic bacteria and *Staphylococcus aureus* are sometimes seen.

Clinical features

These include malaise, fever, a blocked nose with purulent nasal discharge and pain and discomfort on one side of the face associated with headaches. Examination reveals tenderness and sometimes redness over the appropriate sinus.

Sinus radiographs may reveal a fluid level or complete opacification in contrast to the mucosal thickening seen in chronic sinusitis.

Antibiotics

Antibiotics such as aminopenicillins, co-amoxiclav or co-trimoxazole will normally result in rapid improvement, although after several acute attacks chronic sinusitis can occur due to irreversible damage occurring to the sinus mucosa.

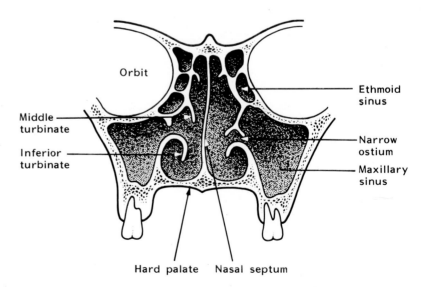

Fig. 3.1 Schematic diagram of the anatomy of the maxillary sinuses.
Note the ostium (arrow) is poorly placed to provide efficient drainage. Reproduced by permission of Baillière Tindall.

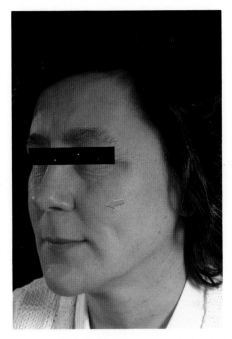

Fig. 3.2 This 38-year-old woman was admitted with symptoms of acute sinusitis that had not settled with a course of oral ampicillin. Redness and tenderness were noted over her maxillary sinus (arrow).

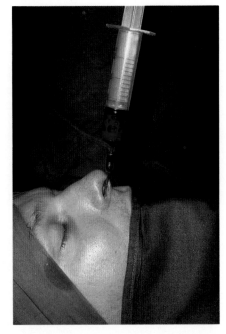

Fig. 3.4 A maxillary sinus puncture and washout was performed under general anaesthesia. Culture of the blood-stained aspirated mucopus revealed a mixed growth of *Haemophilus influenzae* and beta-lactamase-producing *Moraxella catarrhalis*. She made a good recovery with co-amoxiclav antibiotic therapy.

PHARYNGITIS

Although pharyngitis occurs most commonly in conjunction with the common cold or other viral infections, sore throat associated with fever and malaise can be a feature of more serious disease such

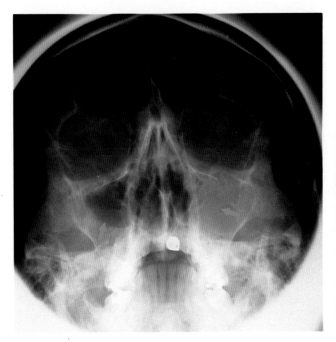

Fig. 3.3 The X-ray showed that her left maxillary sinus was completely opaque (single arrow) and the right had a small fluid level present (double arrows).

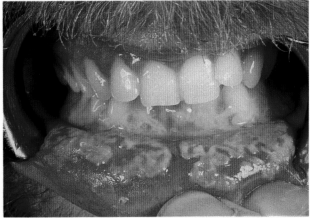

Fig. 3.5 This patient developed marked *Herpes simplex* gingivostomatitis associated with pharyngitis as a first presentation of *Herpex simplex* infection. Rarely, *Herpes simplex* pneumonia can also develop but is usually only seen in immunocompromised individuals.

as streptococcal infection (particularly in primary school children), glandular fever, herpes virus and occasionally *Mycoplasma pneumoniae* infections in young adults.

It is clinically difficult to differentiate a bacterial pharyngitis from that caused by a viral infection such as glandular fever and if antibiotics are prescribed, erythromycin is preferred to an aminopenicillin because of the risk of hypersensitivity rash with the latter.

INFECTIONS OF THE UPPER RESPIRATORY TRACT CAUSING STRIDOR

Such infections can present as a medical emergency due to swelling and obstruction in the pharynx or larynx. Inspiratory stridor is common early in childhood due to the relatively small size of the larynx.

Croup

The most usual cause is acute viral laryngotracheobronchitis (croup). Croup is primarily a disease of children aged between three months and three years and is commoner in boys. The main pathogens are parainfluenza virus, respiratory syncytial virus, influenza virus, rhinovirus and adenovirus. After a few days of upper respiratory tract symptoms, dyspnoea, hoarseness and a deep husky cough develop with evidence of respiratory distress and stridor. Fortunately, most children recover without specific treatment though a small proportion require intubation to protect their airways.

Diphtheria

Although this infection remains a problem in some parts of the world, it is uncommon in developed countries due to immunization programmes. It may still present as a cause of acute airway obstruction.

Epiglottitis

This is an acute, serious infection involving not only the epiglottis but also the arytenoids and the aryepiglottic folds. Although the usual age range of patients is one to six years, over a fifth of those affected are adults. The infection is almost always caused by *Haemophilus influenzae*, type b.

Clinical features

The onset is usually abrupt with fever, toxaemia (which may cause sudden death), marked throat

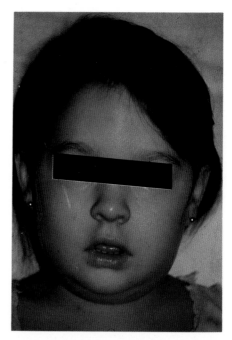

Fig. 3.6   This child presented with fever, nasal discharge, difficulty in breathing and neck swelling. Inflammatory oedema associated with pharyngotonsillar disease resulted in a 'bull neck'.

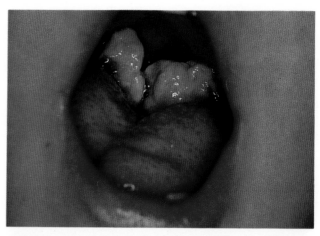

Fig. 3.7   Oral examination revealed an extensive necrotic membrane adherent to the tonsils and adjacent pharynx. The child was one of three infected children, none of whom had been immunized. Treatment with diphtheria antitoxin and erythromycin was curative. Contacts were checked and offered immunization.

pain, dysphagia and respiratory distress. Stridor may be more evident than cough.

Although obtaining a direct view of the epiglottis may be diagnostic, the resulting manipulation may precipitate acute upper airways obstruction. The swollen epiglottis can often be identified on lateral neck radiographs.

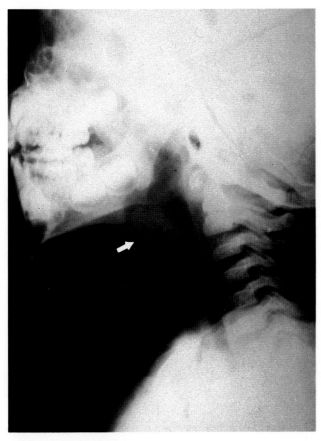

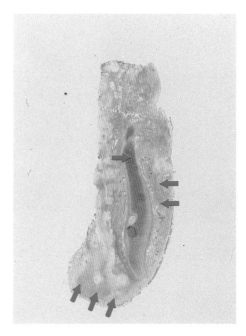

Fig. 3.9 Pathologically, the epiglottis was grossly swollen and acutely inflamed. The cartilage is stained dark blue-red (single arrow) and the soft tissue is grossly swollen with dark-staining inflammatory cells (double arrows) and necrotic slough over the tip (treble arrows).

Fig. 3.8 This is the lateral neck radiograph of a two-year-old child who presented with acute rapidly fatal epiglottitis caused by *Haemophilus influenzae* type b. It shows the swollen epiglottis or 'thumb sign' (arrowed).

Treatment

Management includes recognizing the diagnosis, maintaining an adequate airway, if necessary with intubation, and appropriate antibiotics. Chloramphenicol or a beta-lactamase-stable cephalosporin such as cefotaxime are recommended as initial therapy in view of the problem of ampicillin-resistant *H. influenzae* type b organisms.

FURTHER READING

Arndal, H. and Andreassen, U. K. (1988) Acute epiglottitis in children and adults. Nasotracheal intubation, tracheostomy or careful observations? Current status in Scandinavia. *Laryngologie, Rhinologie Otologie*, **102**, 1012–16.

Behlau, I. and Baker, A. S. (1990) Upper respiratory infections. *Current Opinions in Infectious Diseases*, **3**, 157–65.

Hall, C. B. and McBridge, J. T. (1989) Upper respiratory tract infections. In *Respiratory Infections: Diagnosis and Management*, 2nd edn (ed. J. Pennington), pp. 97–118. Raven Press, New York.

Phelan, P. D. (1991) Respiratory infections in childhood. *Current Opinions in Infectious Diseases*, **4**, 150–4.

4. Community-acquired Pneumonia

INTRODUCTION

Community-acquired pneumonia relates to infections developing out of hospital and either managed at home or being the reason for hospital admission. The incidence in developed countries is said to vary from around three cases per 1000 adult population a year to an annual rate of 10–15 cases per thousand population for all ages, the rate being very much higher in young children and the elderly. Consequently, community-acquired pneumonia causes large numbers of hospital admissions each year and in developing countries pneumonia is the commonest cause of adult hospital attendances.

The majority of community-acquired pneumonias can be treated at home without the need for hospital management; only 20% of cases require admission.

EPIDEMIOLOGY

A knowledge of the epidemiology of common types of community-acquired infection is very helpful for the clinician as some pathogens have characteristic seasonal patterns (Fig. 4.1). Respiratory infections and pneumonia are much commoner during the first quarter of the year, associated with the peak activity of respiratory viruses such as influenza virus. Respiratory syncytial virus (RSV), the commonest cause of childhood lower respiratory infection and bronchiolitis, appears in early and mid-winter.

Bacterial pneumonias, including serious pneumococcal, staphylococcal, *Haemophilus* and *Moraxella* infections, are seen more frequently during periods of influenza virus activity in late winter. For some reason *Haemophilus* infections are also more common in the autumn. *Mycoplasma* infection produces a different pattern. Although endemic cases are somewhat commoner in the autumn, large epidemics

occur throughout the world every three or four years and last about a year, during which time *Mycoplasma* becomes a very prominent cause of chest infections and pneumonia.

ENVIRONMENTAL FACTORS

Most respiratory infections are transmitted from person to person by direct contact or by droplet spread. Thus spread of influenza, *Mycoplasma* infection or whooping cough can often be traced through a family, school or workplace. In contrast, other community-acquired pneumonias are zoonotic or acquired from the environment. *Legionella* infection is the classic example of the latter, where infected water droplets are inhaled by a susceptible host. Many natural and man-made water systems are contaminated with low levels of *Legionella* bacteria, and warm temperatures, contaminants and particulate matter in the water, and stagnant or slow flow, all favour the multiplication of the organisms, which may reach very high numbers. An aerosolized mist of infected droplets can be produced around showers, spray taps, cooling towers, recreational whirlpools and faulty air conditioning units. Infection following inhalation of the infected droplets into the lungs of a susceptible host results in sporadic or epidemic *Legionella* pneumonia.

Figure 4.2 illustrates the problem. The plume or water mist from this cooling tower on a factory site was implicated as a source of a *Legionella* outbreak.

Examples of zoonotic infections include psittacosis, Q fever and tularaemia.

Psittacines and all other species of birds may harbour *Chlamydia psittaci* in their gastrointestinal and biliary systems (Fig. 4.3). The organism is excreted in large numbers at times of stress and illness, when the birds can be highly infectious both

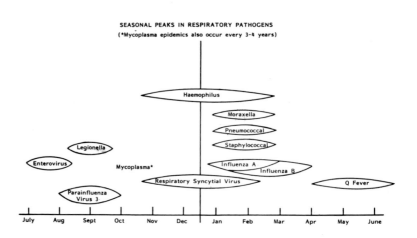

SEASONAL PEAKS IN RESPIRATORY PATHOGENS
(*Mycoplasma epidemics also occur every 3-4 years)

Fig. 4.1 Diagram illustrating usual seasonal peaks of common respiratory pathogens. Reproduced by permission of Baillière Tindall.

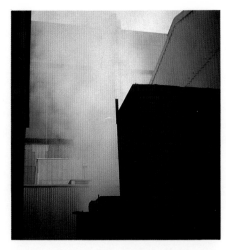

Fig. 4.2   Plume from a cooling tower that was implicated in an outbreak of *Legionella* infection.

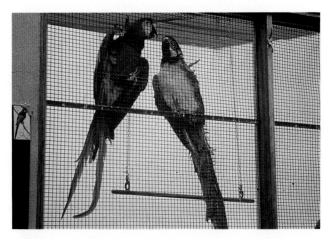

Fig. 4.3   Psittacines and many other species of birds may harbour *Chlamydia psittaci*.

to other birds and to humans. Recently a separate species, *Chlamydia pneumoniae*, has been described without an avian host and with direct human to human spread.

Many animals, in particular sheep and goats, can harbour *Coxiella burnetii*. By-products of conception, such as placental tissue, are particularly liable to be heavily contaminated at lambing time. The organism is very resistant to drying, and infected dust can cause disease, distanced in both time and space from the original infected animal. Similarly, *Francisella tularensis*, the cause of tularaemic pneumonia, is found in nature associated with a large number of wild animals, especially squirrels, rabbits and hares. Most human disease is acquired from contact with infected animals or via deerfly or tick bites. Rarer causes of pneumonias caused by animal-associated infections include anthrax caused by *Bacillus anthra-*

cis, brucellosis pneumonia, plague pneumonia due to *Yersinia pestis*, and *Pasteurella multocida* respiratory infections (also see Chapter 8).

AETIOLOGY

Only a few pathogens cause the large majority of community-acquired pneumonias. Bacteria are the cause in 60–80% of cases, viruses in 10–15% and atypical pneumonias in 10–20%. In this context, atypical pneumonias are defined as those infections that are acquired in the community and do not respond to penicillin antibiotics but do show response to other antibiotics such as the macrolide erythromycin. They include infections caused by *Mycoplasma pneumoniae*, *Chlamydia* species and *Coxiella burnetii*. Community-acquired *Legionella* pneumonia is sometimes included.

A summary of the causes of community-acquired pneumonia as shown in a variety of recent studies is given in Table 4.1.

Pneumococcal infection remains by far the commonest cause, other bacteria being much less common. In the elderly, atypical infections are uncommon. *Haemophilus* infections and, in the very debilitated, Gram-negative bacillary pneumonias can

Table 4.1   Causes of adult community-acquired pneumonia

	Incidence (%)
Bacterial	
Strep. pneumoniae	30–70
H. influenzae	5–12
Legionella pneumophila	3–5
Staph. aureus	1–3
Moraxella catarrhalis	0–1
Gram-negative bacilli	Rare
Other bacteria	Rare
Atypical	
Mycoplasma pneumoniae	3–18
Chlamydia species	2–3
Coxiella burnetii	1–2
Viruses	
Influenza virus	5–10
Other viruses	5–8
No cause found	30–50

occur. In contrast, in children under two years, the major lower respiratory infection is RSV bronchiolitis. In neonates, streptococcal, staphylococcal, Gram-negative and chlamydial infections are seen.

CLINICAL FEATURES

No pathogen has a presentation sufficiently unique to allow its early differentiation from the other causes of pneumonia. However, in general, bacterial infections tend to develop more quickly, be associated with more signs of general toxaemia, have more prominent physical signs in the chest, be more commonly associated with homogeneous shadowing on the chest radiograph and have a raised blood leucocyte count. In contrast, atypical infections such as *Mycoplasma* pneumonia tend to have a more insidious onset, affect younger people, run a milder course and may have more extensive radiographic shadowing than would be thought likely from physical examination of the chest. Unfortunately there is considerable overlap, making a definitive clinical diagnosis of the cause of the pneumonia impossible.

CLINICAL APPROACH TO MANAGEMENT

The cause of the pneumonia is generally not known at the time that the clinician needs to decide about antibiotic therapy. Fortunately, the relatively few causes of community-acquired pneumonia make a logical antibiotic choice relatively easy. Epidemiological clues do influence the choice. Any antibiotic chosen must provide effective cover against pneumococcal infection, by far the commonest

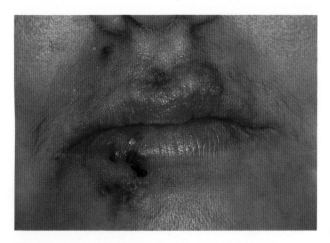

Fig. 4.4 Herpes labialis is seen particularly with pneumococcal pneumonia.

cause. An aminopenicillin is often a good choice with erythromycin a sensible alternative in penicillin-allergic patients and also appropriate if an atypical or *Legionella* infection is suspected. Newer macrolides such as clarithromycin and azithromycin are also likely to be very valuable in this setting. In the presence of chronic lung disease *Haemophilus influenzae* and *Moraxella catarrhalis* are possible agents; an aminopenicillin, co-amoxiclav, co-trimoxazole or a newer generation oral cephalosporin or macrolide are appropriate antibiotics. Qunolones can be helpful where initial antibiotics have been ineffective or contraindicated by hypersensitivity or toxic reactions.

GENERAL MANAGEMENT

In addition to antibiotics the general management of the patient is particularly important in those with moderate or severe infection. Such patients should be recognized early and those with serious infection investigated and monitored carefully. Adequate oxygen therapy and fluid management is essential for such patients, who should be observed closely and transferred to an intensive care unit if and when necessary. Assisted ventilation may be required for advancing respiratory failure and can be life saving.

SPECIFIC BACTERIAL INFECTIONS

Pneumococcal pneumonia

The classical clinical presentation of pneumococcal pneumonia is with abrupt onset of fever, rigors, pleural chest pain, and cough with rusty-coloured sputum. Chest examination may reveal bronchial breathing from lobar consolidation but more usually inspiratory crepitations. Herpes labialis is seen in up to a third of patients and is commoner than with other types of pneumonia (Fig. 4.4).

The chest radiograph in Fig. 4.5 displays the typical features with dense homogeneous consolidation in one or more lobes; in this case in the right middle lobe and apex of the right lower lobe.

The initial stage in the pathogenesis is of congestion followed by alveolar exudate rich in fibrin and red blood cells (red hepatization) and then grey hepatization when numerous polymorphs fill the alveoli. The cause of the radiographic appearances can be appreciated when examining the lung from a fatal case of bacteraemic pneumococcal pneumonia with the left lower lobe showing uniform consolidation or grey hepatization without any loss of

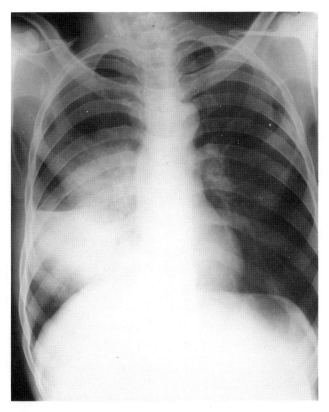

Fig. 4.5   Chest radiograph of a man with pneumococcal pneumonia showing homogeneous consolidation in right middle lobe and apex of right lower lobe.

Fig. 4.6   Lung of a woman who died of left lower lobe pneumococcal pneumonia. Note the pale consolidated lobe without loss of volume or purulent material in the bronchi.

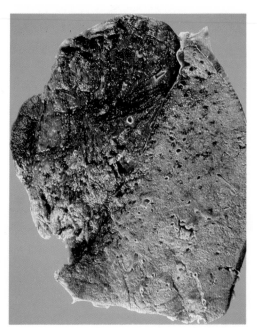

volume. Note the absence of purulent material in the bronchi (Fig. 4.6).

A microphotograph of the lung, at the stage shown in Fig. 4.6, shows alveoli uniformly filled with fibrin and inflammatory cells which are mostly polymorphonuclear leucocytes. The alveolar walls are preserved and undamaged (Fig. 4.7).

Although a sympathetic pleural effusion can develop in about a quarter of cases with pneumococcal pneumonia, infection of the fluid is less common, occurring in around 1%.

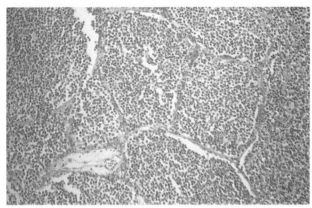

Fig. 4.7   Microphotograph of section of consolidated lung (from Fig. 4.6) showing alveoli filled with inflammatory cells but with intact alveolar walls.

Fig. 4.8   In this case a 24-year-old man presented with an eight-day history of pneumococcal pneumonia, complicated by a large pericardial effusion and left pleural empyema. Two litres of pus were drained from the pericardial space. Reproduced by permission of Baillière Tindall.

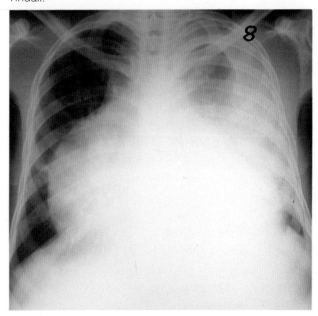

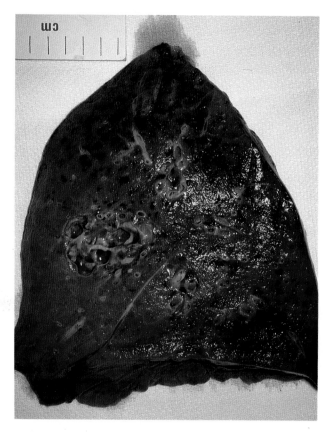

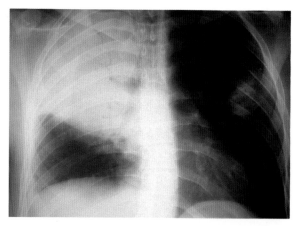

Fig. 4.11 In this case, a 19-year-old man was admitted with a two-day history of high fever, right pleural pain and cough with blood-stained sputum following a week of a 'flu-like' illness. *Streptococcus pneumoniae* serotype 3 was grown from his sputum and blood cultures.

Fig. 4.9 Local lung necrosis and abscess formation is unusual with pneumococcal pneumonia but occurred in this consolidated lung of a 72-year-old man who died of the more virulent type 3 pneumococcal infection.

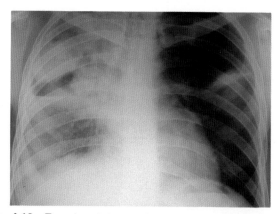

Fig. 4.12 Two days later, cavitation occurred within his right upper lobe consolidation and he coughed up purulent sputum.

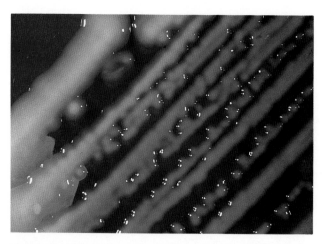

Fig. 4.10 Shiny mucoid colonial appearance of *Streptococcus pneumoniae* serotype 3 on blood agar.

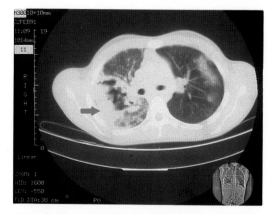

Fig. 4.13 A CT chest scan confirmed the extensive cavitation within his right upper lobe (arrow). He gradually improved with prolonged penicillin therapy. Follow-up serological tests confirmed a recent influenza A virus infection which increased the severity of his pneumococcal infection.

Streptococcus pneumoniae serotype 3 is a particularly virulent strain which on blood agar produces an extremely mucoid colonial appearance which reflects the large quantity of capsular polysaccharide material that is produced (Fig. 4.10).

In most cases resolution of the histological appearances is complete with return to structural normality. Late complications of pneumococcal pneumonia are uncommon but can include organization of exudate into lung fibrosis.

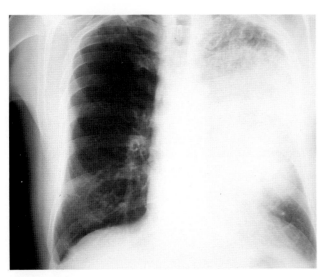

Fig. 4.14 A 72-year-old man with chronic obstructive bronchitis presented with bacteraemic pneumococcal pneumonia.

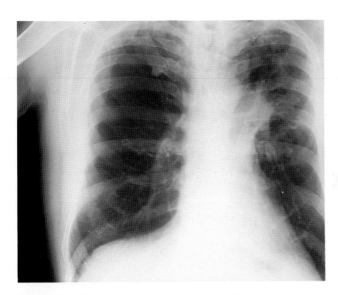

Fig. 4.15 Although he made a full clinical recovery, four months later his chest radiograph shows contraction and fibrotic lines in the left upper zone following his severe pneumococcal infection. Bronchoscopy was normal.

Other streptococcal pneumonias

Streptococcus pyogenes, a beta-haemoloytic streptococcus, can be the cause of severe pneumonia in children and young adults, often following a viral infection. Enzymes and haemolysins are produced which enhance pathogenicity so that abscess formation and early empyema are not uncommon.

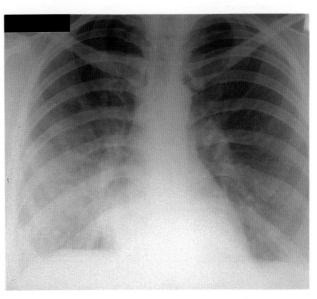

Fig. 4.16 A 27-year-old mother developed the symptoms of acute bacterial pneumonia preceded by 10 days of flu-like symptoms. The chest radiograph showed extensive right-sided consolidation and a pure, heavy growth of *Streptococcus pyogenes* was cultured from both sputum and bronchial aspirates. Serological tests showed evidence of recent *Mycoplasma* infection and she responded to high dose penicillin therapy.

Staphylococcal pneumonia

Pneumonia caused by *Staphylococcus aureus* is most commonly seen as a complication of primary influenza virus infection. Following the influenzal illness, the patient appears to be recovering but then becomes unwell with fever, toxaemia, purulent (often blood-stained) sputum and signs of pneumonia. The chest radiograph may show features suggestive of staphylococcal pneumonia such as cavitating consolidation of a lobe (Fig. 4.17).

In the presence of staphylococcal bacteraemia, disseminated infection can occur in the lung with multiple discrete areas of consolidation with abscess formation occurring (Fig. 4.18).

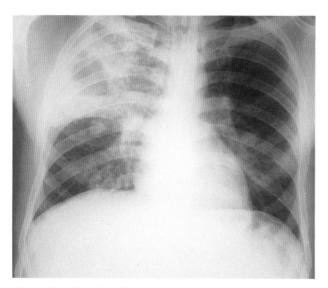

Fig. 4.17 Chest radiograph of staphylococcal pneumonia showing cavitation and consolidation.

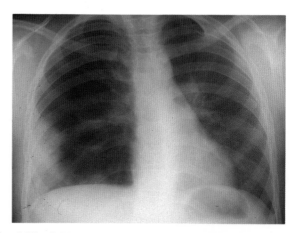

Fig. 4.19 A 58-year-old man presented with right middle lobe consolidation and a pure, heavy growth of *Staphylococcus aureus* was cultured from his sputum.

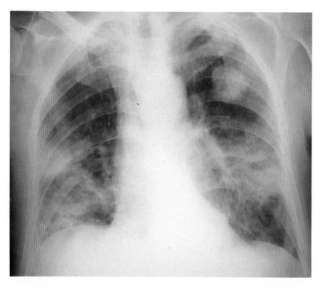

Fig. 4.18 Multiple discrete areas of consolidation with abscess formation are seen on the chest radiograph of a 68-year-old man with bacteraemic staphylococcal pneumonia.

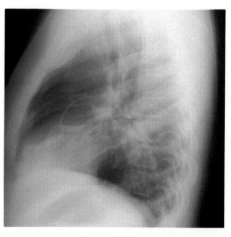

Fig. 4.20 A lateral chest radiograph clearly shows two pneumatocoeles (arrows) with small fluid levels which are also apparent on the PA view shown in Fig. 4.19.

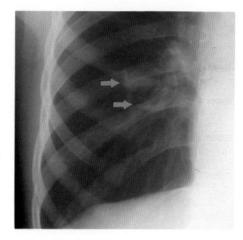

Fig. 4.21 Two months later, following antibiotic therapy, the consolidation had resolved but the pneumatocoeles are still visible (arrows).

Acute tension cysts or pneumatocoels are occasional features, particularly in infection in childhood. They probably occur due to a ball valve effect in diseased bronchioles. They are also seen in adults on occasion.

As regards diagnosis, at least 25% of cases will have positive blood cultures. Sputum smears can be helpful in over two-thirds of cases and provide a rapid indication of the likely cause of the pneumonia.

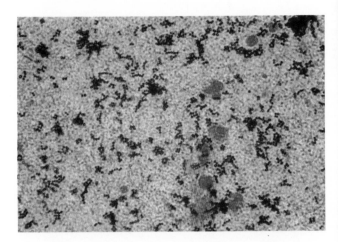

Fig. 4.22 This Gram stain of expectorated sputum from a previously well 37-year-old engineer who developed a secondary severe pneumonia following an attack of influenza A infection demonstrates pus cells and numerous Gram-positive cocci in clumps, which were confirmed to be *Staphylococcus aureus* on culture.

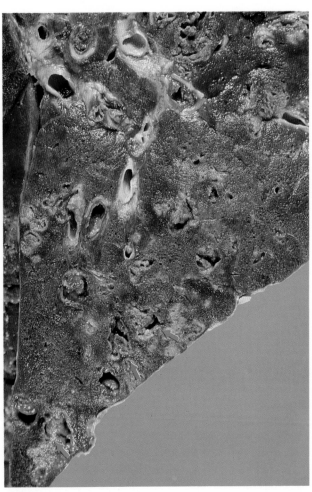

Fig. 4.24 Multiple abscesses can be seen on the close-up view (arrow).

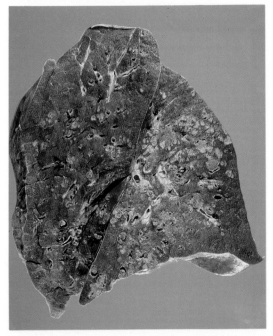

Fig. 4.23 His condition deteriorated rapidly in spite of full medical management and assisted ventilation. At post mortem, widespread consolidation and abscess formation was present.

GRAM-NEGATIVE BACTERIAL PNEUMONIA

Moraxella catarrhalis

Moraxella catarrhalis is a Gram-negative diplococcus formerly called *Branhamella catarrhalis*. It is a commensal of the upper respiratory tract but has been implicated in cases of pneumonia in patients with underlying lung disease though it is also cultured from the sputum of about 4% of adults with bronchitis. Its importance is that around half of the strains produce beta-lactamase.

volved and there is nothing specific about the clinical features of *Haemophilus* pneumonia. Radiographically, the pattern is normally a patchy basal bronchopneumonia similar to that found with *Moraxella catarrhalis* (see Fig. 4.25).

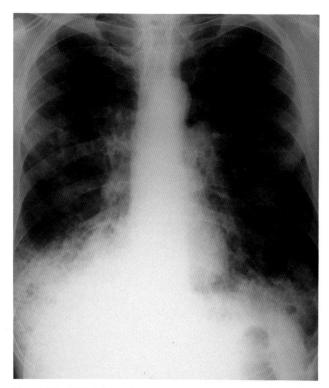

Fig. 4.25 This is the chest radiograph of a 70-year-old man with chronic obstructive bronchitis and a patchy right lower lobe pneumonia. He did not improve with amoxycillin.

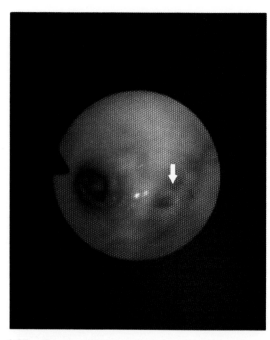

Fig. 4.27 This bronchoscopic photograph of a 74-year-old smoker being investigated for a left lung bronchophenumonia shows the features of acute bronchitis with red inflamed bronchial mucosa and pus in the left main bronchus (arrow), from which *H. influenzae* was cultured.

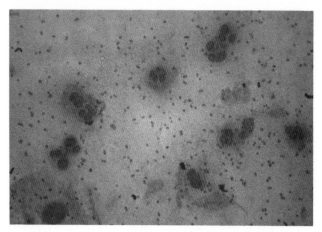

Fig. 4.26 Gram stain of his sputum demonstrated the typical appearance of *Moraxella catarrhalis*, confirmed to be a beta-lactamase-producing strain on culture. He recovered with co-amoxiclav therapy.

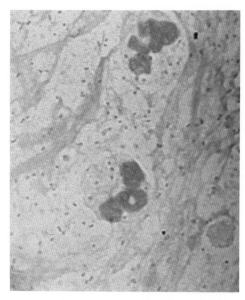

Fig. 4.28 Gram stain of *H. influenzae* in sputum, revealing weakly staining Gram-negative coccobacilli.

Haemophilus influenzae

H. influenzae is increasingly recognized as a cause of bacterial pneumonia, as well as bronchitis in adults, particularly in those with underlying chronic lung disease. Non-capsulated strains are normally in-

Electron microscopy of the organism can confirm the pleomorphic nature of *H. influenzae* with its marked variation in size and shape (Fig. 4.29).

An aminopenicillin is the drug of choice for susceptible strains. However, there is increasing ampicillin resistance of about 8% in the UK and higher in other parts of Europe such as Spain, and also in the USA. Alternative effective agents include co-amoxiclav, co-trimoxazole, quinolones and later generation cephalosporins.

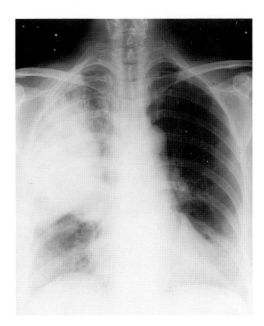

Fig. 4.30 A 40-year-old woman had recently returned from a holiday hotel in the Mediterranean. She had a four-day history of fevers, rigors, aches and pains, severe headache, dry cough and dyspnoea. The development of confusion had precipitated her hospital admission. This chest radiograph shows extensive homogeneous consolidation of the right upper lobe and patchy changes in the right lower lobe.

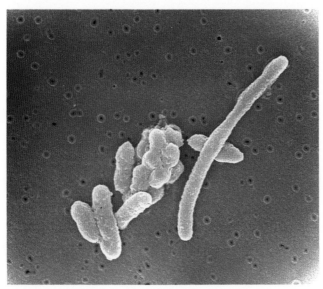

Fig. 4.29 Electron micrograph of *H. influenzae* confirming pleomorphic nature of the organism. Division is taking place within the organism at the centre of the field.

Legionella infections

Legionella pneumophila is a short stubby flagellated Gram-negative bacillus that will not grow on ordinary media and takes a Gram stain poorly. *Legionella* pneumonia is commoner in men, with the highest incidence in 40–70-year-olds. The incubation period is up to 14 days after exposure to a source of infected water droplets and clinical presentation can vary from a mild respiratory illness to fulminating pneumonia.

The organism grows best on buffered charcoal yeast extract (BCYE) agar, having a typical glistening colonial appearance. (Fig. 4.33).

Histologically the characteristic picture of *Legionella* pneumonia is of alveoli filled with a mixed inflammatory cell content of mononuclear cells with some polymorphs. The alveolar walls are preserved (Fig. 4.34).

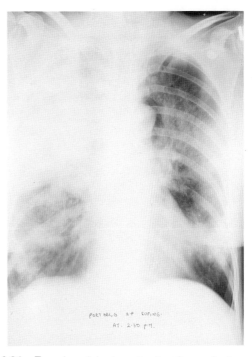

Fig. 4.31 Two days later her chest radiograph shows extensive spread of the pneumonia in spite of intravenous ampicillin and erythromycin. She required assisted ventilation.

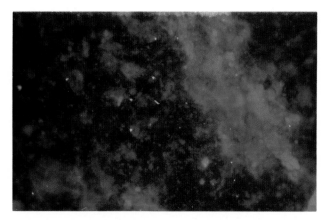

Fig. 4.32 Direct immunofluorescent staining of bronchial aspirates was positive for *Legionella pneumophila* serogroup I, with the organisms appearing as bright rods and dots amongst background debris. The diagnosis was subsequently confirmed by repeat serological testing.

A silver stain of the alveolar exudate can be used to demonstrate numerous small slender silver-positive *Legionella* organisms, many of which are intracellular (Fig. 4.35).

An electron micrograph of an infected white cell shows many *Legionella* organisms intracellularly inside phagosomes (Fig. 4.36). This is one explanation why only a few antibiotics appear to be effective in this disease as they require the ability to penetrate into the vacuoles in the inflammatory cells where the organism is dividing. Erythromycin remains the treatment of choice; there is anecdotal evidence that quinolones such as ciprofloxacin and rifampicin are also effective.

The mortality of *Legionella* pneumonia is around 12% but lower in previously fit patients. In survivors, clinical and radiographic recovery can be slow

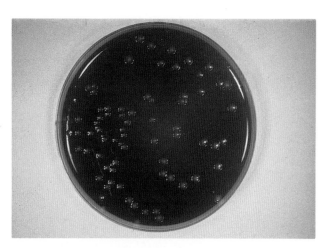

Fig. 4.33 Typical glistening colonial appearance of *Legionella pneumophila* on buffered charcoal yeast extract agar.

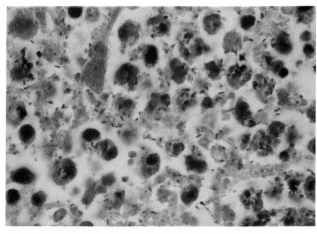

Fig. 4.35 *Legionella* organisms can be identified by silver staining and show up as small slender intracellular silver-staining rods within the alveolar exudate.

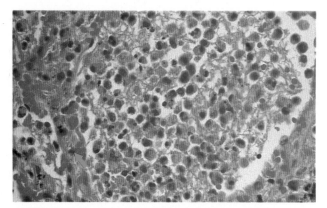

Fig. 4.34 Characteristic histological features of legionella pneumonia with preserved alveolar walls (arrow) and a mixed inflammatory cell alveolar exudate.

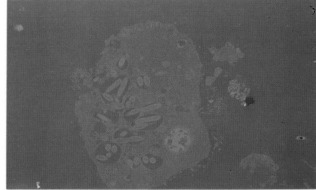

Fig. 4.36 An electron micrograph of an infected white cell showing many intracellular *Legionella* organisms within vacuoles. Reproduced by permission of Baillière Tindall.

and radiographs may take many months to clear. Residual permanent, fibrotic lines are not unusual (Fig. 4.37).

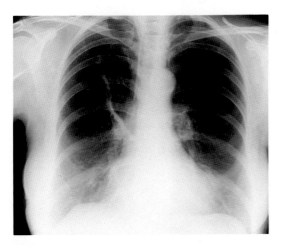

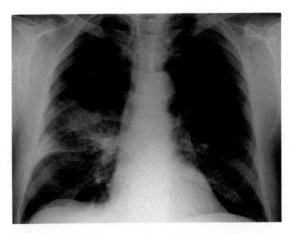

Fig. 4.39 *Klebsiella pneumoniae* was isolated from the blood and sputum of a 49-year-old alcoholic who was admitted with a one-week history of pneumonia, toxaemia and haemoptysis. He was treated successfully with cefotaxime.

Fig. 4.37 Residual fibrotic lines in the right upper lobe of same patient as in Fig. 4.30, three months after clinical recovery from *Legionella* pneumonia.

Gram-negative bacillary infections

Although aerobic Gram-negative bacillary infections are frequently the cause of nosocomial pneumonia, they are much less common as a community infection, occurring usually in very debilitated individuals. Examples are shown in Figs 4.38 and 4.39.

Pasteurella multocida is a small Gram-negative coccobacillary organism that can cause pneumonia in individuals with chronic lung disease, particularly bronchiectasis and lung cancer. The organism is usually acquired from animals and is also seen as a frequent cause of cat and dog cellulitis. Lower lobe infection is usually seen, sometimes with abscess or empyema formation, and the sputum is usually purulent. An example of this infection is shown in Figs 4.40–4.45.

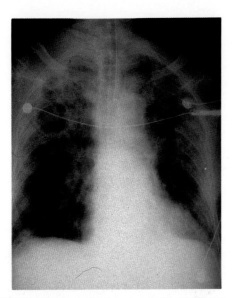

Fig. 4.38 An elderly patient was admitted with fulminating septicaemic community-acquired *Pseudomonas aeruginosa* pneumonia. She had been a resident in a nursing home and had received several courses of antibiotics for chest infections over the previous four weeks.

Fig. 4.40 These series of pictures were taken from a 48-year-old woman with long-established bilateral cystic bronchiectasis. Her chest radiograph in 1984 showed changes in the left lower zone and right mid-zone.

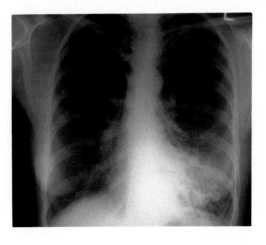

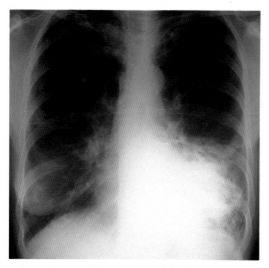

Fig. 4.41 Her condition was considerably worse during 1990 and 1991, with a dramatic increase in her production of purulent sputum.

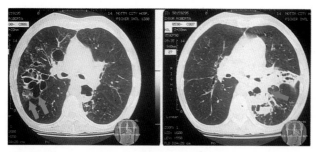

Fig. 4.42 Extensive consolidation and pus-filled cysts are well seen on a CT scan in her left lower lobe (single arrow). Cystic bronchiectasis can be seen in her right lung (two arrows).

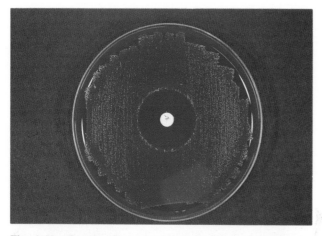

Fig. 4.43 *Pasteurella multocida* was repeatedly isolated from her sputum in spite of long-term high dose penicillin therapy. Colonies can be seen growing on blood agar plate with a well-defined zone of growth inhibition around a penicillin disk.

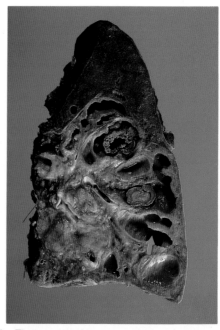

Fig. 4.44 The resected lung specimen confirmed extensive lung destruction and suppuration with grossly dilated bronchi (arrow).

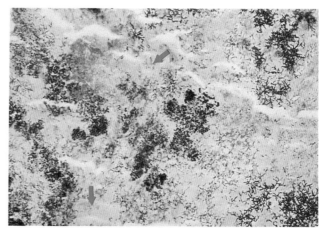

Fig. 4.45 A Gram stain of the necrotic debris within the cysts revealed a mixture including large numbers of Gram-negative bacilli (arrow) confirmed to be *Pasteurella multocida* on culture.

ATYPICAL PNEUMONIAS

Mycoplasma pneumonia

Mycoplasma pneumoniae mostly affects schoolchildren and young adults. It is a cause of both upper and lower respiratory infections and only a small proportion will develop pneumonia. The type of pneumonia can be very variable. In up to half of adults homogeneous segmental or lobar consolidation similar to bacterial pneumonia occurs (Fig. 4.46).

Histologically, *Mycoplasma* pneumonia is characterized by extensive interstitial inflammatory infiltrate of mononuclear cells, mostly lymphocytes and plasma cells, with sparse alveolar exudate (Fig. 4.49) and is associated with a marked and at times suppurative bronchiolitis which may lead to bronchiolitis obliterans (Fig. 4.50).

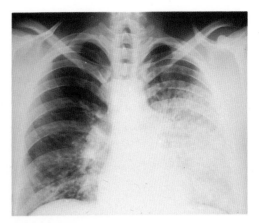

Fig. 4.48   A patient with *Mycoplasma* pneumonia was initially treated with ampicillin but the chest radiograph five days later showed extensive bilateral homogeneous and patchy consolidation. The patient made a good recovery with erythromycin.

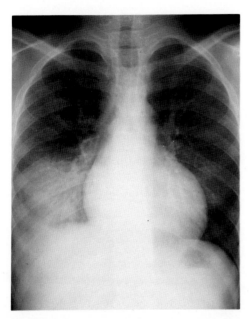

Fig. 4.46   Homogeneous consolidation on the chest radiograph of a patient with *Mycoplasma* pneumonia.

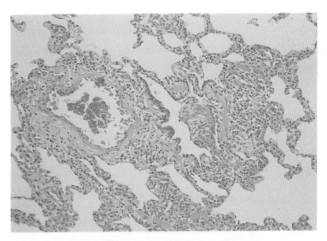

Fig. 4.49   Histological appearances of acute *Mycoplasma* pneumonia with extensive interstitial infiltrate (arrow) and sparse alveolar exudate.

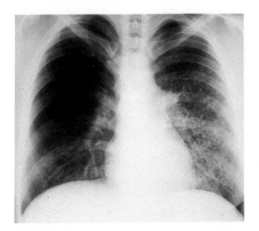

Fig. 4.47   The initial chest radiograph of a 28-year-old patient demonstrates the more usually recognized radiographic pattern with patchy left-sided infiltrates. *Mycoplasma pneumoniae* infection was confirmed serologically in paired serum samples.

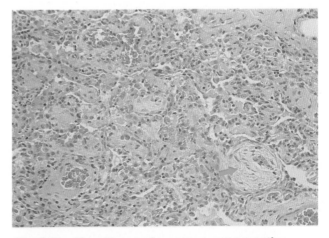

Fig. 4.50   *Mycoplasma* also causes a suppurative bronchiolitis which may lead on to bronchiolitis obliterans (arrow).

Mycoplasma pneumoniae infection can sometimes present with prominent non-respiratory symptoms and signs. Various rashes can occur, including the Stevens-Johnson syndrome, as shown by the marked ulceration of the lips in a patient with severe

of blood are added to a prothrombin tube which is cooled in a 4°C fridge. Coarse agglutination confirmed the presence of cold agglutinins in the blood of a 20-year-old student subsequently proven serologically to have mycoplasma pneumonia (Fig. 4.54).

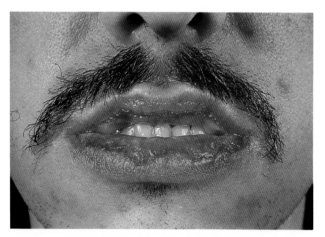

Fig. 4.51   Stevens–Johnson syndrome associated with *Mycoplasma* **pneumonia.**

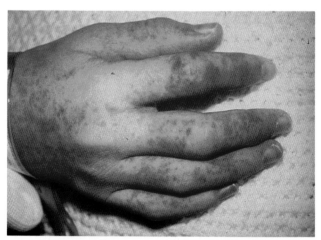

Fig. 4.53   Although cold agglutinins are common with *Mycoplasma pneumoniae* **infection, cold agglutinin peripheral ischaemia is an unusual complication.**

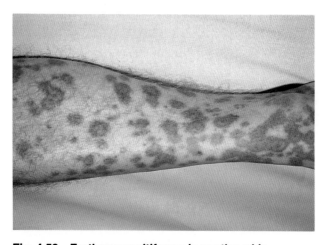

Fig. 4.52   Erythema multiforme is another skin manifestation of *Mycoplasma* **infection.**

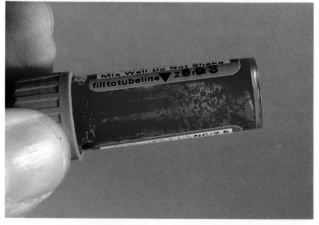

Fig. 4.54   Coarse agglutination of blood confirms the presence of cold agglutinins in the bedside cold agglutinin screening test.

mycoplasma pneumonia (Fig. 4.51). A patient with extensive erythema multiforme caused by mycoplasma infection is shown in Fig. 4.52.

About a half of patients produce cold agglutinins in their blood at some stage during their illness. Occasionally this can cause clinical problems, either from haemolytic anaemia or from cold agglutinin peripheral ischaemia (Fig. 4.53).

Detecting the presence of cold agglutinins can be used as a useful, quick diagnostic test. A few drops

Psittacosis

The epidemiology of *Chlamydia psittaci* infection has already been discussed. The clinical presentation varies from a mild influenza-like illness to a fulminating multi-system toxic state. The latter is explained by the haematogenous spread which occurs to the lung and elsewhere during the late incubation period of the infection. Common symptoms include high fever, shivers, headache, myalgia and a dry cough. The patient is often confused and toxic and the clinical picture can be similar to that of *Legionella* pneumonia. The white blood count is usually normal. Shadowing on the chest radiograph is usually patchy, involving a lower lobe initially although spread can occur.

The pathological features of psittacosis are illustrated in Figs 4.56–4.58.

Characteristic inclusion bodies can be seen in tissue culture preparations, in Fig. 4.59 stained by an immunofluorescent techique.

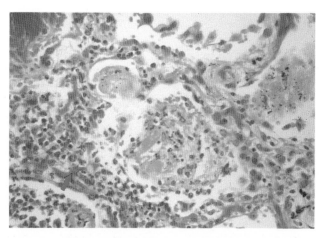

Fig. 4.57 Histologically there is congestion of alveolar walls (arrow) and fibrin together with a largely mononuclear cell infiltrate in the alveolar spaces.

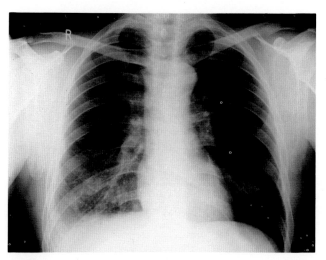

Fig. 4.55 Patchy right lower lobe pneumonia is seen in the chest radiograph of this woman with psittacosis whose husband, a pet shop owner, had recently acquired several psittacine love birds, one of whom he brought home as a house pet.

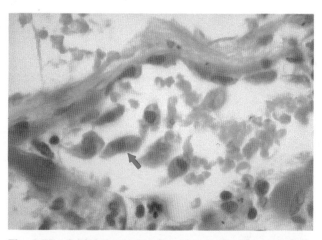

Fig. 4.58 A higher power view shows the characteristic features of psittacosis pneumonia with desquamation of swollen alveolar lining cells (arrow) resulting in the name 'alveolar cell pneumonia'.

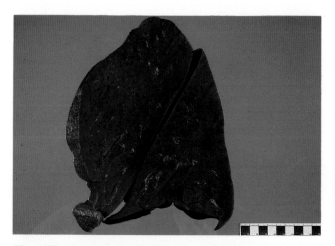

Fig. 4.56 A whole lung slice of a fatal case of psittacosis shows a congested, rather solid, appearance generally.

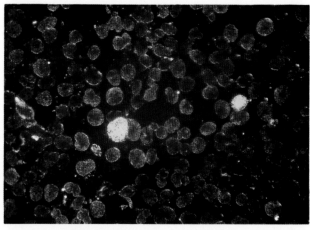

Fig. 4.59 Characteristic inclusion bodies can be seen in tissue culture preparations stained by an immunofluorescent technique.

Q fever

There are no specific or radiographic features of *Coxiella burnetii* pneumonia and the presentation is usually mild and similar to *Mycoplasma* infection. Chronic Q fever infection can result in endocarditis.

RESPIRATORY VIRUSES

Influenza virus

Influenza virus is the commonest respiratory virus to cause disease. There are three types (A, B, C) determined by their internal nuclear protein. Most disease is caused by type A (Fig. 4.60).

The brunt of the infection is borne by the columnar epithelial cells of the respiratory tract which are penetrated and destroyed, resulting in denudation of the tracheobronchial ciliated epithelium with associated severe hyperaemia and haemorrhage. This is illustrated in a necropsy specimen of the tracheobronchial tree of a man who died of influenza A infection complicated by acute staphylococcal bronchopneumonia (Fig. 4.61).

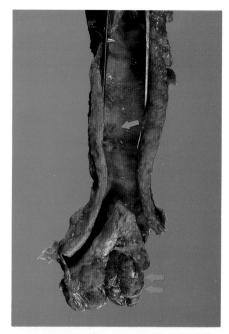

Fig. 4.61 Tracheobronchial tree of a 70-year-old man who died of influenza A infection complicated by acute staphylococcal bronchopneumonia. Note the haemorrhagic and purulent tracheobronchitis (one arrow). The subcarinal lymph nodes are reactively enlarged (two arrows).

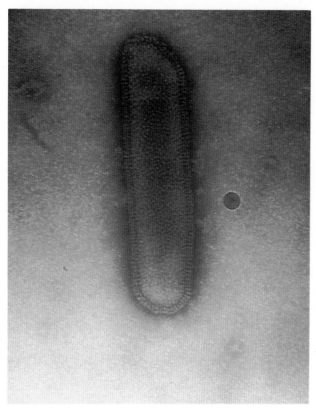

Fig. 4.60 Electron micrograph of influenza virus type A.

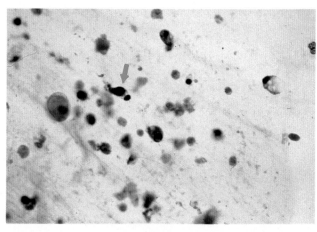

Fig. 4.62 Expectorated respiratory epithelial cells which have lost their cilia and have became cuboidal (arrow) as a result of influenza virus infection.

Giemsa stain of the sputum from a patient with influenzal pneumonia reveals shedding of respiratory epithelial cells which have lost their cilia and become cuboidal (Fig. 4.62). In contrast, a similar stain on normal expectorated sputum shows the presence of normal ciliated respiratory epithelial cells (Fig. 4.63).

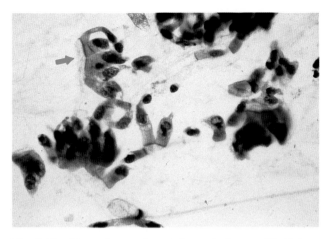

Fig. 4.63   Normal expectorated respiratory epithelial cells are ciliated and columnar (arrow).

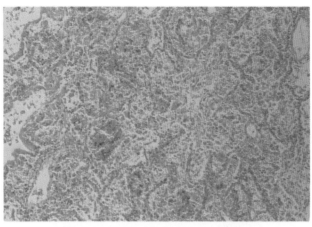

Fig. 4.65   Haemorrhagic consolidation of the lung from a fatal case of primary influenza pneumonia.

Primary influenza pneumonia is less common than a secondary bacterial pneumonia. In the former, the symptoms of the pneumonia merge with the influenzal illness, crackles are heard in the lung and the chest radiograph shows diffuse progressive bilateral infiltrates.

In fatal cases the pathological picture is usually of haemorrhagic pneumonic consolidation (Fig. 4.65). High power views show alveolar septa infiltrated by mononuclear cells with fibrinous exudate in alveolar spaces (Fig. 4.66).

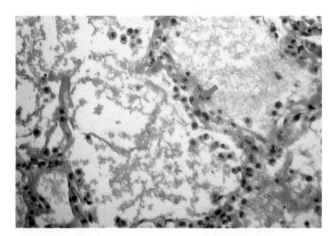

Fig. 4.66   Histologically the features of influenza pneumonia include mononuclear cell interstitial infiltration (arrow) and fibrinous exudate in alveolar spaces.

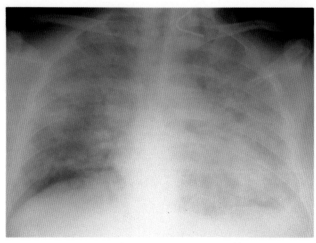

Fig. 4.64   Diffuse progressive bilateral infiltrates are shown on the radiograph of a 36-year-old man who presented with proven influenza B pneumonia. No bacterial pathogens were found in his sputum, bronchial aspirates or blood and there was no response to antibiotics. He made a gradual recovery with supportive therapy and received a short period of treatment nebulized with ribavirin.

Measles virus pneumonia

Worldwide, measles is a major cause of morbidity and mortality among children. The typical rash and clinical presentation of measles with conjunctivitis of mucosal involvement is well known (Fig. 4.67).

Pneumonia may occur early in the infection, often as a result of secondary bacterial infection in malnourished children or as a viral 'giant cell' pneumonia developing three or four weeks after exposure to measles. The diffuse pneumonia frequently progresses and prognosis remains poor. The typical histological appearance is of mononuclear inflammatory cells and fibrin filling the alveolar spaces and alveolar walls and giant cells formed by transformation of the alveolar lining cells (Fig. 4.68).

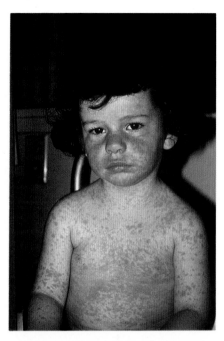

Fig. 4.67   Typical features of measles infections with rash and mucosal inflammation.

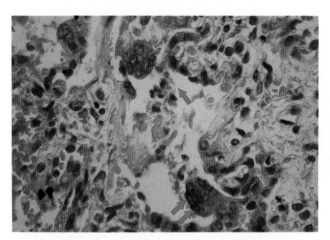

Fig. 4.68   Typical histological features of measles pneumonia with alveoli and alveolar walls filled by exudate and mononuclear cells (one arrow) together with giant cells (two arrows).

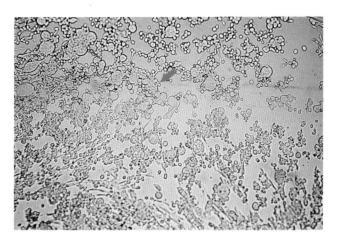

Fig. 4.69   RSV growing in tissue culture causing syncytial formation in some areas (arrow).

The child presents with bronchiolitis which can be severe. There is now therapy available for severe cases in the form of aerosolized ribavirin, an antiviral agent. Administration is via a small particle aerosol generator 'SPAG' which can produce a continuous mist of aerosolized drug into a transparent box over the baby's head (Fig. 4.70).

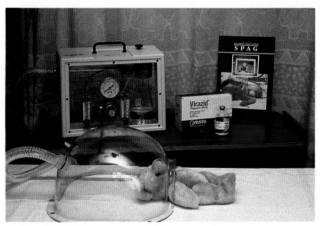

Fig. 4.70   Transparent head box used to deliver aerosolized ribavirin to babies with severe RSV infection.

RSV infection

RSV infection is the commonest viral respiratory pathogen in infants. It acquired its name from the typical cytophathic effect of the virus on HEp2 cells in tissue culture. The normal architecture is severely disrupted, with swelling of cells, and in some areas there is syncytial formation as illustrated in Fig. 4.69.

Adenovirus infections

Adenoviruses are important causes of both upper and lower respiratory infections in children, causing pneumonia, croup and bronchiolitis as well as pharyngitis and pharyngoconjunctival fever. An electron micrograph of adenovirus particles obtained from a child with conjunctivitis is shown in Fig. 4.71

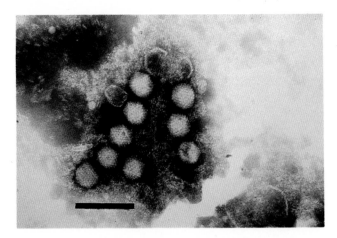

Fig. 4.71 Electron micrograph of adenovirus particles showing the typical icosahedral shape. The bar equals 100 μm.

and reveals the typical symmetrical icosahedral morphology of the nucleocapsid.

The pneumonic consolidation is characteristically necrotic but not suppurative with progressive destruction of alveolar walls (Fig. 4.72).

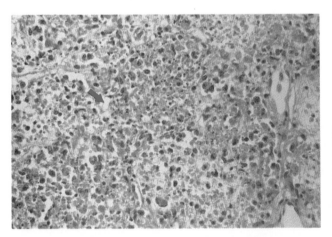

Fig. 4.72 Adenovirus pneumonia characteristically is associated with destruction of alveolar walls (arrow).

Herpes virus infections

Varicella-zoster can cause severe pneumonia in adults. Following an incubation period of up to 21 days, respiratory symptoms can develop shortly after the rash with cough, dyspnoea and chest pains and progressive bilateral fluffy infiltrates on the chest radiograph (Fig. 4.73–4.75).

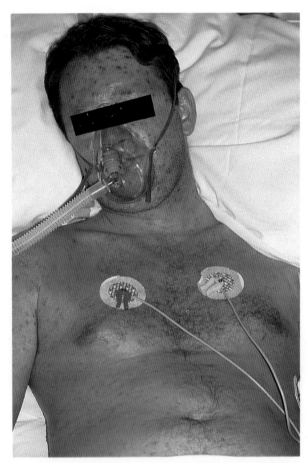

Fig. 4.73 This 28-year-old father acquired chicken-pox from his daughter and was admitted with acute respiratory distress.

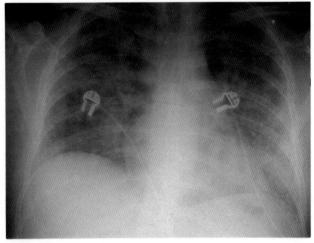

Fig. 4.74 His chest radiograph showed extensive bilateral fluffy shadowing consistent with *Varicella* pneumonia. He required a short period of assisted ventilation but made a rapid recovery with intravenous acyclovir.

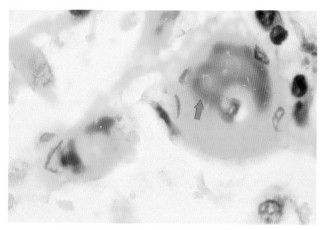

Fig. 4.77 Inclusion bodies (arrow) seen within degenerate pneumocytes in *Varicella-zoster* pneumonia (phloxine tartrazine stain).

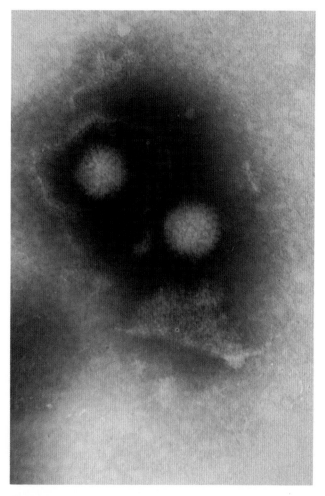

Histologically, the characteristic finding is a mild interstitial mononuclear cell infiltrate and degenerative cytopathic changes in the much swollen alveolar pneumocytes (Fig. 4.76).

A phloxine tartrazine stain can be used to demonstrate that the degenerative pneumocytes contain cytoplasmic inclusion bodies (Fig. 4.77).

In survivors, recovery is normally complete, although scattered calcification can be seen on follow-up radiographs, being commoner in cigarette smokers (Fig. 4.78).

Fig. 4.75 Electron microscopy of fluid obtained from a vesicle on the patient's skin showed the morphological characteristics of the herpes virus with an irregular envelope surrounding the nucleocapsid.

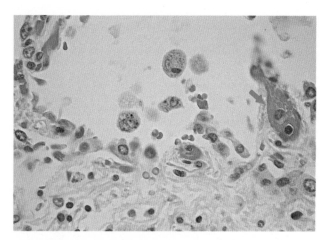

Fig. 4.76 The characteristic histological features of *Varicella-zoster* pneumonia include interstitial mononuclear cell infiltrate with swollen alveolar pneumocytes (arrow).

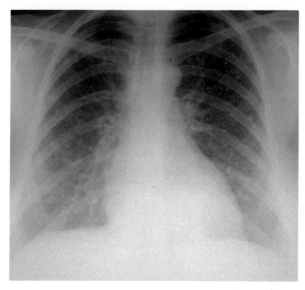

Fig. 4.78 Punctate calcification is shown scattered throughout the lung fields on the chest radiograph of this 30-year-old female cigarette smoker who had had chickenpox pneumonia eight years previously.

FURTHER READING

British Thoracic Society, Public Health Laboratory Service (1987) Community acquired pneumonia in adults in British hospitals in 1982–83: a survey of aetiology, mortality, prognostic factors and outcome. *Quarterly Journal of Medicine*, **239**, 195–200.

Glynn, J. R. and Jones, A. C. (1990) Atypical respiratory infections. *Current Opinion in Infectious Diseases*, **3**, 169–75.

Macfarlane, J. T. (1987) Community acquired pneumonia. *British Journal of Diseases of the Chest*, **81**, 116–27.

Pennington, J. E. (ed.) (1989) *Respiratory infections: Diagnosis and Management*. Raven Press, New York.

Shale, D. J. (ed.) (1991) Respiratory infections. *Current Opinion in Infectious Diseases*, **4**, 131–76.

5. Hospital-acquired Pneumonia

INTRODUCTION

Hospital-acquired (nosocomial) pneumonia is common and adds considerably to the morbidity of any primary illness requiring hospital management. As such it is an important cause of death. The pathogenesis of nosocomial pneumonia is multifactorial and reflects both host vulnerability and microbial virulence.

PATHOGENESIS

Host factors include advanced age, chronic cardio-pulmonary disease, malignancy, chronic renal failure and progressive neurological disease, especially where consciousness is impaired or pharyngeal reflexes are compromised. Postoperative patients are particularly at risk, especially where anaesthesia has been prolonged or a period of postoperative ventilation has been necessary; patients within an intensive care unit are among the most at risk of developing nosocomial pneumonia. The increasing use of cytotoxic and immunosuppressive drugs, including corticosteroids, in the management of malignant and non-malignant disease has increased the risk of pneumonia, especially in patients in whom neutrophil function is comprised or neutropenia is present.

Aspiration of oropharyngeal secretions is common both in health and disease but is aggravated by ill health, impaired consciousness, endotracheal and nasogastric intubation, as well as neurological disturbance of the normal protective reflex mechanisms and gastro-oesophageal disease. The microbial aetiology of hospital-acquired pneumonia is summarized in Table 5.1. In contrast with the aetiology of community-acquired pneumonia, there is a relative increase in Gram-negative bacillary pathogens such as *Klebsiella pneumoniae* and *Pseudomonas aeruginosa* as well as *Staphylococcus aureus*. Not only are infections caused by these pathogens intrinsically more virulent but the choice of antibiotic therapy is more limited and differs from those used to treat community-acquired infection. *Legionella pneumophila* infection must also be considered as a cause of nosocomial infections where it results either in epidemic or sporadic infection. Other occasional bacterial pathogens include *Haemophilus influenzae* and *Streptococcus pneumoniae* since these may persist as part of the upper respiratory tract flora.

Hospitalization is associated with changes in the distribution of the respiratory bacterial flora. Microorganisms are acquired from other patients and in particular staff, who act as vehicles for microbial transmission. Other sources include shared medicaments and topical applications, while food may transmit selected pathogens such as *Klebsiella* and *Serratia* spp. Changes in the bacterial flora can occur within a few days of admission, particularly in high dependency units. This in part explains the greater predominance of Gram-negative bacillary infections within intensive care unit (ICU) patients where antibiotic use provides an additional pressure that encourages the emergence of a Gram-negative flora. Several of these issues are now illustrated.

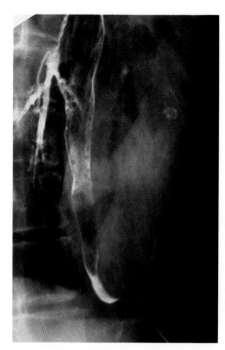

Fig. 5.1 The pathogenesis of aspiration pneumonia is well illustrated by an elderly male patient who was under investigation for dysphagia. A barium swallow produced a simultaneous bronchogram due to extrinsic obstructive lesion of the oesophagus which was subsequently shown to be caused by a laryngeal carcinoma. Two days after this radiographic examination, the patient developed the typical features of a right basal pneumonia. The cause of the aspiration was quite obvious in this patient.

Other gastro-oesophageal causes such as hiatus hernia and motility disorders should also be considered. Inhaled lipid material 'floating' in the stomach due to delayed emptying may complicate the pneumonic reaction by causing an exogenous lipid pneumonia (see also Chapter 7). Aspiration may present acutely with pneumonia, as in the case described, but in other patients may result in lung abscess (see Chapter 7) and in part reflects the less virulent nature of oropharyngeal anaerobic bacteria which predominate in lung abscess.

Table 5.1 Microbial aetiology of hospital-acquired pneumonia

Common

Pseudomonas aeruginosa
Staphylococcus aureus
Klebsiella pneumoniae

Less common

Enterobacter spp.
Serratia marcescens
Escherichia coli
Proteus spp.
Acinetobacter spp.
Aspergillus spp.
Haemophilus influenzae
Anaerobic bacteria
Streptococcus pneumoniae

Occasional

Legionella pneumophila
Viruses

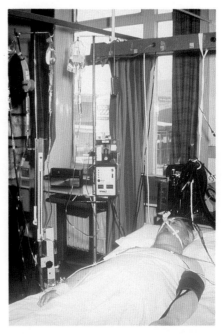

Fig. 5.3 Patients admitted to intensive care units are especially vulnerable to nosocomial pneumonia. Normal host defences are impaired through mechanical support systems and nosocomial bacterial flora rapidly colonize the oropharynx which is the major source of such infections.

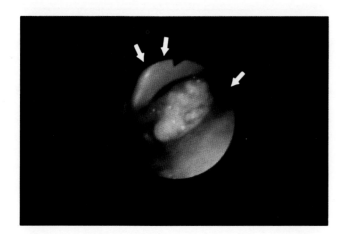

Fig. 5.2 An 80-year-old man was admitted with a large supraglottic tumor (one arrow) seen at endoscopy behind the epiglottis (two arrows). He had increasing dysphagia together with coughing and choking after food. He developed aspiration pneumonia with abscess formation from which a mixture of anaerobes and Gram-negative bacilli were obtained on fine needle aspiration.

Patients within ICUs (Fig. 5.3) are particularly at risk of hospital-acquired pneumonia. Prolonged ventilation impairs the normal physiological protective mechanisms of warming, humidification and particle filtration of inspired air. The requirement for regular mechanical bronchial toilet, owing to the absence of normal mucociliary clearance, predisposes to aspiration of upper airways secretions. Nasogastric intubation further compromises the situation. The use of H_2 antagonists and other pH modulators has been linked with an increase in bacterial numbers within gastro-oesphageal and pharyngeal secretions, and an increased frequency of pneumonia. The opportunities for cross-infection are also substantial within the ICU, owing to the high staff/patient ratio and the frequent requirement for hand contact in the maintenance and monitoring of vital functions.

EXAMPLES OF HOSPITAL-ACQUIRED PNEUMONIA

Figure 5.4 is the chest radiograph of an elderly patient who developed *Pseudomonas aeruginosa* pneumonia in the ICU five days after emergency surgery for a perforated peptic ulcer. The diagnosis was established by positive blood cultures in addition to repeatedly positive cultures of respiratory secretions. He was treated with a combination of ceftazidime and gentamicin to which he made a good response. Unfortunately there is a high mortality associated with *Pseudomonas aeruginosa* pneumonia.

Figure 5.5 illustrates the post mortem appearances

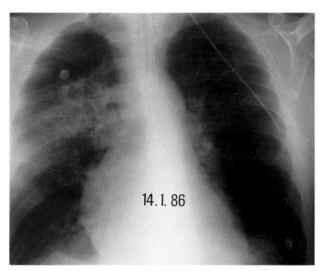

Fig. 5.4 Acute cavitating right upper lobe ***Pseudomonas aeruginosa*** **pneumonia in a man receiving assisted ventilation on intensive care unit.**

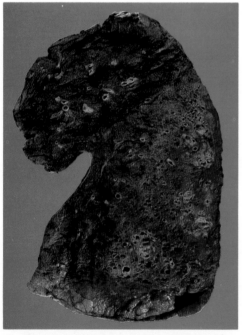

Fig. 5.5 ***Pseudomonas aeruginosa*** **pneumonia demonstrating extensive abscess formation in areas of pneumonic consolidation of the lower lobe.** When freshly sliced this pus is much greener in colour.

in another patient. This demonstrates a multifocal suppurative pneumonia. The purulent abscess contents usually have a characteristic green colour when freshly incised.

Occasionally, 'outbreaks' of hospital-acquired pneumonia occur. When caused by *Legionella*

pneumophila, infection is often linked to a common source such as a contaminated air conditioning system, or hot and cold water supply systems which can cause infection by droplet inhalation from contaminated showers. Other pathogens may cause epidemic clusters of infection and suggest a common source.

Figure 5.6 shows a corrugated rubber Y piece used in the ventilation of patients during oesophageal surgery. Over a 10-day period three patients undergoing surgery within a thoracic unit developed postoperative *Pseudomonas aeruginosa* pneumonia within 48 hours of their operation. This early onset pneumonia, occurring as a cluster of cases, suggested a common source. The Y piece was found to contact *Ps. aeruginosa* which was similar in type to the outbreak strain. On investigation it was discovered that the Y piece was being simply washed in tap water at the end of each operation and hung up to dry; the moisture remaining within the corruga-

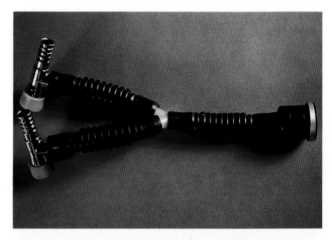

Fig. 5.6 Y-connector anaesthetic tubing used in oesophageal surgery. Inadequate sterilization led to colonization with *Pseudomonas aeruginosa* and an outbreak of early postoperative pneumonia in four patients requiring oesophageal surgery. Samples from the tubing and sputum showed all isolates to be identical.

tions provided an ideal culture environment for *Pseudomonas*. The simple expedient of sterilizing the piece of equipment brought the epidemic to a halt.

Klebsiella pneumoniae is another cause of serious Gram-negative pneumonia. It has the ability to produce an extremely destructive necrotizing pneumonia with abscess formation. Mortality is high.

Figure 5.7 shows the chest radiographic appearance of a patient with *Klebsiella pneumoniae* pneumo-

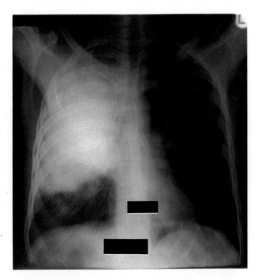

Fig. 5.7 Community-acquired right upper lobe *Klebsiella* pneumonia with 'swollen' lobe and drooping horizontal fissure.

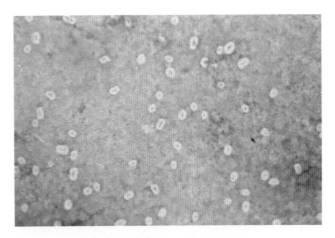

Fig. 5.9 India ink preparation of *Klebsiella pneumoniae*. Note clear zone around each organism which reflects the abundant capsular material of this pathogen.

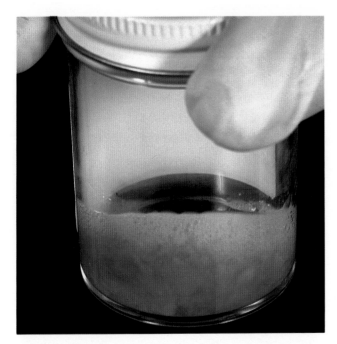

Fig. 5.8 Browny haemorrhagic sputum from a patient with cavitating pneumonia caused by *Klebsiella pneumonias* (see Fig. 5.10).

nia. The patient was a long-standing alcoholic and when admitted was extremely unwell. His sputum was copious and brick red in colour as shown in Fig. 5.8. On sputum microscopy large numbers of pus cells will be visible, together with Gram-negative bacilli which, after isolation, were examined by the India ink technique to demonstrate encapsulation

(Fig. 5.9); the capsule is one of the major virulence factors of this pathogen.

On occasion, *Klebsiella pneumoniae* infection may produce chronic cavitating lung disease as in Fig. 5.10. Antibiotics should be selected carefully when treating these infections since klebsiellae are normally resistant to ampicillin. Treatment relies on an aminoglycoside, often in combination with a broad-spectrum cephalosporin such as cefotaxime.

In the newborn, Gram-negative bacillary pneumonia may also complicate hospitalization. It has a poor prognosis and is often fatal despite appropriate antibiotic treatment. Figure 5.11 illustrates the post mortem appearance of a newborn child who dies from *Escherichia coli* pneumonia. Both lungs show

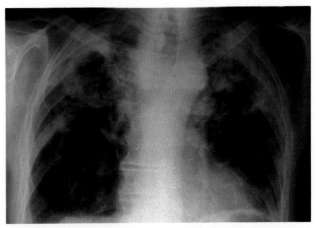

Fig. 5.10 Chest radiograph showing bilateral upper lobe consolidation and cavitation due to chronic *Klebsiella* pneumonia.

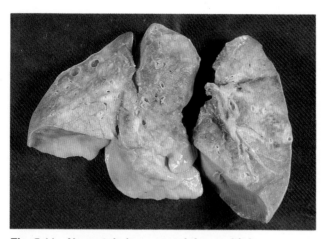

Fig. 5.11 **Neonate's lung containing multiple abscesses (arrows) due to *Escherichia coli* complicating upper respiratory tract infection.**

multiple abscesses due to aspiration of infected upper respiratory tract material.

The emphasis in all these varieties of nosocomial pneumonia is early recognition, prompt and appropriate antibiotic therapy together with judicious ventilation, supplemented with careful fluid and electrolyte balance. Prevention is obviously desirable and regrettably not sufficiently considered. The importance of avoiding cross-infection by hand-washing is obvious but too often ignored, while careful bronchial toilet in the ventilated can reduce the risk of aspiration lung infection.

FURTHER READING

Craven, D. E. and Driks, M. R. (1987) Nosocomial pneumonia in the intubated patient. *Seminars in Respiratory Infection*, **2**, 20–33.

Driks, M. R., Craven, D. E., Bartolome, R., Celli, B. R., Manning, M., Burke, R. A., Garvin, G. M., Kunches, L. M., Farber, H. W., Wedel, S. A. and McCabe, W. R. (1987) Nosocomial pneumonia in intubated patients given sucralfate as comared with antacids or histamine type 2 blockers. *New England Journal of Medicine*, **317**, 1376–82.

Kinnear, W. J. M., Finch, R. G., Pilkington, R. and Macfarlane, J. T. (1990) Nosocomial lower respiratory tract infections in surgical wards. *Thorax*, **45**, 187–9.

Korvick, J. A., Yu, V. L. and Fang, G. (1987) Legionella species as hospital-acquired respiratory pathogens. *Seminars in Respiratory Infection*, **2**, 34–47.

Levison, M. E. and Kaye, D. (1985) Pneumonia caused by gram-negative bacilli: an overview. *Review of Infectious Diseases*, **7S**, 656–65.

Pennington, J. E. (1990) Nosocomial respiratory infection. In *Principles and Practice of Infectious Diseases*, 3rd edn (eds F. L. Mandell, R. G. Douglas Jr. and J. E. Bennett), pp. 2199–205. John Wiley and Sons, New York.

6. Lung Disease in the Immunocompromised and HIV-infected host

INTRODUCTION

The immunocompromised host presents an increasing and challenging medical problem. Such patients are vulnerable to a wide spectrum of infections which frequently involve the respiratory tract. The immunocompromised state may be short-lived or life-long and includes true states of immunodeficiency, as well as immunosuppression from acquired disease or therapeutic intervention. Host defences are affected in many ways. The physical barriers of skin and mucous membranes may be compromised by cytotoxic drugs as well as the use of intravascular and bladder catheters. The inflammatory response may be variably affected either from a relative absence of, or poorly functioning, granulocytes and macrophages, while a variety of humoral mediators of protection can be downregulated by disease or chemotherapy. Immunodeficiency states include the relatively uncommon congenital defects of cell-mediated or humoral immunity and the numerically more frequent states of acquired immunodeficiency. Only a brief discussion of these immunodeficiency problems is appropriate for the purpose of illustrating the patterns of respiratory disease that may ensue.

Hyposplenism may result from surgical removal or congenital absence, or secondary to a haemoglobinopathy, e.g. sickle cell disease. It predisposes to serious infection, especially from organisms such as *Streptococcus pneumoniae*, since opsonic antibody activity is impaired. Multiple myeloma is likewise associated with a defiency of humoral immunity and frequently presents with a respiratory infection since an abnormal paraprotein production is at the expense of normal immunoglobulins.

Cell-mediated immune function is frequently disturbed by the wasting which accompanies malignant disease. The lymphomas and chronic lymphocytic leukaemia are most clearly linked with impaired cell-mediated immune function which is also compromised by the use of high dose corticosteroid therapy. In recent years the emergence of human immunodeficiency virus (HIV) infection has emphasized the spectrum of disease linked to acquired impairment of cell-mediated immunity. By selectively targeting the CD4 lymphocytes, HIV results in a series of opportunistic infections and unusual malignancies which define the natural history of the acquired immunodeficiency syndrome.

Phagocytic activity may also be impaired as a result of an absolute deficiency or impaired phagocyte function. Neutropenia is most usually seen in association with a variety of haematological malignancies and brought about by cytotoxic chemotherapy. It is well recognized that when the absolute neutrophil count falls below $0.5 \times 10^9/l$, episodes of infection increase substantially, especially with sustained counts below $0.1 \times 10^9/l$. With bone marrow recovery immunosuppression resolves.

In this brief discussion of the immunocompromised host the emphasis has been on defined immunodeficiency and immunosuppressive problems. However, the general issues of impaired host defences as they apply to the respiratory tract and which have been discussed in Chapter 5 are particularly important to the populations referred to in this section.

PNEUMOCYSTIS CARINII

Pneumocystis carinii has emerged as the single most important infectious complication of HIV disease and is the major indicator that the disease has progressed to AIDS. Pneumocystosis has been recognized for many years is association with profound malnutrition. However, before the emergence of HIV, *P. carinii* pneumonia (PCP) occasionally complicated organ transplant recipients, acute and chronic lymphocytic leukaemia, the lymphomas and those on high does corticosteroid therapy. In its most characteristic form PCP is accompanied by fever, progressive shortness of breath, cough which is often unproductive, and progressive bilateral alveolar infiltrates largely affecting the lower zones and radiating out from the hila on the chest radiograph. Pleural effusions are uncommon. Hypoxaemia is usual and untreated PCP carries a high mortality. Early treatment with either high dose co-trimoxazole or pentamidine, in those intolerant of the former, is effective. Relapses may occur, especially in those with AIDS, in whom life-long chemoprophylaxis is recommended.

Pneumocystis carinii is generally considered to be a protozoon but recent reports based on genetic analysis suggest that it may be reclassified among the fungi. Its life cycle is illustrated in Fig. 6.1. It is thought that many individuals become asymptomatically infected in early life; disease occurs only in those who subsequently develop profound cell-mediated immunosuppression.

Figure 6.2 is the chest radiograph of a patient with classical *P. carinii* pneumonia (PCP). He was under treatment with high dose corticosteroids and cyclophosphamide for Wegener's granulomatosis.

Figure 6.3 is the radiograph of a patient with more florid disease. He had had a kidney transplant some five weeks earlier.

The diagnosis of PCP should be suspected in the

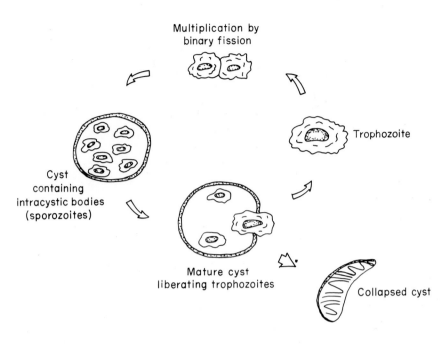

Multiplication by
binary fission

Fig. 6.1   Life cycle of
Pneumocystis carinii.

Trophozoite

Cyst
containing
intracystic bodies
(sporozoites)

Mature cyst
liberating trophozoites

Collapsed cyst

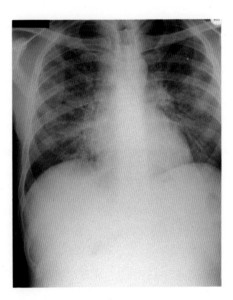

Fig. 6.2   Increased haziness in perihilar areas on chest radiograph due to early *Pneumocystis carinii* infection in a 40-year-old man on immunosuppressive therapy for Wegener's granulomatosis.

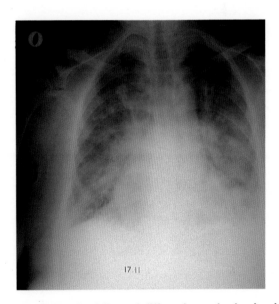

Fig. 6.3   Extensive bilateral diffuse lung shadowing in a patient on immunosuppression following a renal transplant. *Pneumocystis carinii* identified in bronchoalveolar lavage.

presence of the usual clinical and radiographic features and the correct clinical setting.

Figure 6.4 illustrates the early radiographic changes in a patient with HIV infection. In approximately 15% of confirmed cases the chest radiograph is normal at presentation, the clue being unex-plained dyspnoea and hypoxaemia. Additional radiographic support for the diagnosis can be gained from an isotope gallium scan, which produces a characteristic pattern (Fig. 6.5).

Whenever possible, it is desirable to establish a microbiological diagnosis; if the clinical diagnosis is

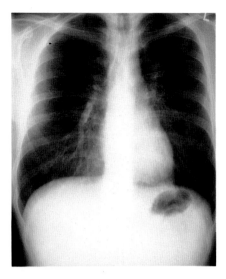

Fig. 6.4 The early chest X-ray appearances of *Pneumocystis carinii* pneumonia. Note the diffuse bilateral infiltrate primarily affecting the lower lung fields and radiating out from the hila. The patient had AIDS.

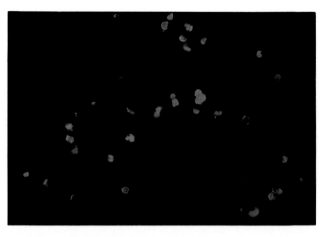

Fig. 6.6 Bronchoalveolar lavage washings stained with methenamine silver. A clump of *Pneumocystis carinii* is visible with typical morphology. The patient had undergone renal transplantation six weeks earlier and had developed progressive hypoxaemia and bilateral lower zone infiltrates unresponsive to conventional antibiotics. He recovered with high dose co-trimoxazole.

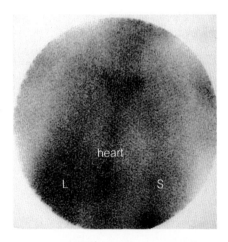

Fig. 6.5 A positive gallium scan in a patient with *Pneumocystis carinii* pneumonia complicating AIDS. Note the diffuse uptake throughout both lung fields as well as within the liver (L) and spleen(S). The cardiac silhouette (arrow) is superimposed on these areas of uptake.

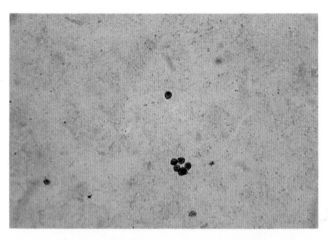

Fig. 6.7 Numerous *Pneumocystis carinii* in centrifuged bronchoalveolar lavage fluid using a fluorescein-labelled monoclonal antibody. The sample was obtained from the patient illustrated in Fig. 6.4.

incorrect the delay in specific therapy and the unnecessary use of high dose and potentially toxic agents can be harmful. The possibility of mixed lung infection must also be kept in mind. Currently, bronchoalveolar lavage (BAL) examination for the presence of *P. carinii* by cytological or immuno-fluorescent techniques is preferred. Figure 6.6 is an example of lavage fluid which has yielded character-istic silver-staining material, while Fig. 6.7 is mate-rial positive for *P. carinii* by immunofluorescence using a monoclonal antibody. The latter technique can also be positive in expectorated sputum but the sensitivity of this method is inferior to BAL-obtained specimens. In practice, spontaneous sputum pro-duction is uncommon in *P. carinii* pneumonia and the sputum often has to be induced with nebulized hypertonic saline (see Chapter 1).

Despite better recognition, fatalities are still com-mon and are the result of overwhelming disease, delayed diagnosis or inadequate therapy. Trans-

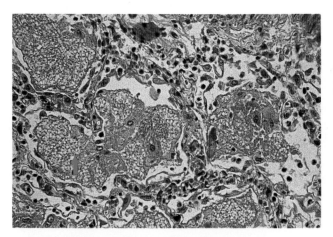

Fig. 6.8 Typical 'foamy' alveolar exudates in *Pneumocystis* **infection as seen in haemotoxylin and eosin sections (arrow).**

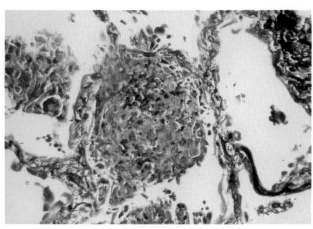

Fig. 6.10 In some more chronic cases of *Pneumocystis carinii* **infection granulomas may form, arousing the suspicion of tuberculous infection.** The true nature can only be identified by silver stains demonstrating the parasite.

bronchial or open lung biopsy material may be necessary to demonstrate characteristic histological appearances of foamy alveolar exudate on haematoxylin and eosin staining (Fig. 6.8) and organisms with methenamine silver preparations (Fig. 6.9). After treatment, degenerate forms and granulomas (Fig. 6.10) may cause diagnostic difficulty for the unwary. At post mortem affected lungs have a pale grey solid mucoid cut surface. Although primarily a disease of the lungs, disseminated *P. carinii* infection has been increasingly reported in those suffering from HIV disease in whom atypical presentations may occur in response to low dose chemoprophylactic regimens.

ASPERGILLOSIS

Aspergilli are saprophytic fungi. The genus includes many species, among which *Aspergillus fumigatus* and to a lesser extent *A. niger* are more prone to produce human disease. Figure 6.11 shows the typical fruiting head of *A. fumigatus*. The myriad of spores readily become airborne, explaining why this fungus is ubiquitous. Spores can be readily demonstrated in the environment, including hospital air, by the use of a settle plate (Fig. 6.12). This consists of a fungal agar plate which is exposed for several hours and subsequently incubated; numerous colonies of *A. fumigatus* are visible. This particular sample was

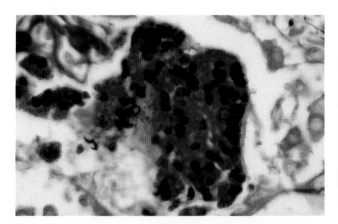

Fig. 6.9 *Pneumocystis carinii* **(Gomori methenamine silver) to show the parasites in the alveolar exudate.** Some cystic forms are present (arrow), while others are more degenerate due to treatment.

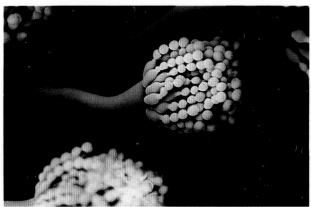

Fig. 6.11 Scanning electron micrograph of the fruiting heads of *Aspergillus fumigatus.* Note the rows of conidia (spores). Magnification × 700.

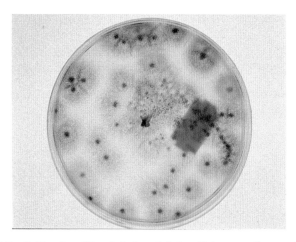

Fig. 6.12 A settle plate (containing Sabouraud's agar) which has been left exposed for six hours in a bone marrow transplant ward. Following incubation for three days, numerous colonies of *Aspergillus fumigatus* are visible. Occasional outbreaks of *Aspergillus* pneumonia have been recognized in severely immunocompromised patients, especially if neutropenia is present.

obtained from air in a bone marrow transplant unit where an outbreak of pulmonary aspergillosis was occurring. The spore size is such that they can be inhaled and reach the alveoli where they may cause disease in the immunocompromised.

A. fumigatus has the ability to produce a fascinating spectrum of human disease which ranges from simple colonization of mucosal surfaces to more extensive proliferation in chronic tuberculous cavities (aspergillomata) and also includes type 1 and type 3 hypersensitivity diseases, which manifest as extrinsic asthma and bronchopulmonary aspergillosis respectively. Profoundly immunocompromised patients, especially those rendered severely neutropenic by chemotherapeutic management of haematological malignancy or for the purposes of bone marrow transplantation, are at special risk from invasive pulmonary aspergillosis. This often disseminates to involve multiple organs and has a high mortality rate. Examples of bronchopulmonary aspergillosis and aspergillomata will be found in Chapters 9 and 12. Aspergillosis of the severely immunocompromised is included in this section.

Invasive pulmonary aspergillosis is the most serious manifestation of *Aspergillus* lung disease. It is most commonly seen in the setting of haematological malignancy or bone marrow transplantation where episodes of profound and prolonged neutropenia (granulocyte count $< 0.1 \times 10^9/l$) render the patient particularly vulnerable to inhaled spores. Most infections are caused by *A. fumigatus*. The early states of the infection are often clinically silent but as

disease advances fever unresponsive to conventional antibiotics occurs. Respiratory symptoms are often absent or limited to an irritating cough. By the time radiographic changes are visible there is usually extensive lung involvement. Although often unilateral initially, bilateral infection is common. The necrotizing process frequently results in cavity

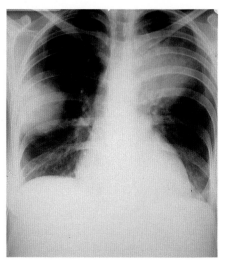

Fig. 6.13   This is a chest radiograph of a patient with acute myeloid leukaemia made neutropenic by chemotherapy. Three weeks into her course of treatment she developed fever and subsequently an unproductive cough. Progressive bilateral radiographic infiltrates became visible. Sputum examination was unhelpful but bronchoscopy with lavage yielded *Aspergillus fumigatus*. She was treated with amphotericin B and improved once bone marrow recovery occurred.

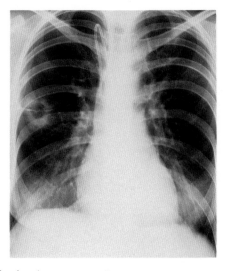

Fig. 6.14   A subsequent radiograph several months later showed significant resolution of the radiographic changes, with the exception of a residual cavity.

formation while the propensity for vascular invasion leads to dissemination in other organs such as the brain, liver and kidneys.

A common clinical problem in neutropenic patients is that of undiagnosed fever. Figure 6.15 shows the temperature chart of such a patient. Despite intensive investigation and broad-spectrum

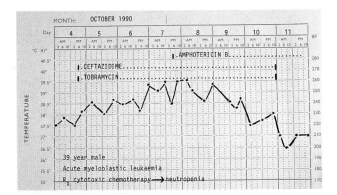

Fig. 6.15 Temperature chart of patient made neutropenic as a result of chemotheraphy for acute myeloblastic leukaemia. The fever was unresponsive to broad-spectrum antibiotics but settled with the addition of intravenous amphotericin B.

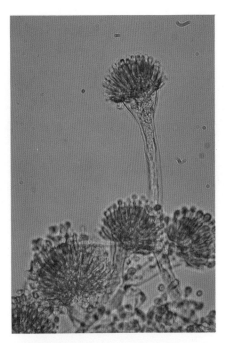

Fig. 6.16 *Aspergillus fumigatus* **from bronchoalveolar lavage material in a patient with neutropenia following bone marrow transplantation.** The culture has been stained with lactophenol cotton blue to demonstrate the typical morphology of the fruiting heads. Magnification × 1000.

antibiotic therapy the fever continued and only fell in response to intraveneous amphotericin B, which targets a broad spectrum of fungal infections in this population. This includes mucosal candidosis, disseminated candida and other yeast infections, as well as the early subclinical manifestations of aspergillosis and other filamentous fungal infections. The precipitin response to *A. fumigatus* is generally absent and therefore repeated isolation of this fungus on sputum examination or in bronchscopic lavage material should raise the suspicion of active infection. Figure 6.16 shows the typical morphology of *A. fumigatus* isolated from lavage material and stained with lactophenol cotton blue.

All too often patients with invasive pulmonary aspergillosis succumb to their infection, especially if bone marrow recovery is delayed. The post mortem appearances are illustrated as follows. The lesions seen in the lung in the invasive disease are necrotic (Fig. 6.17), commonly subpleural (Fig. 6.18) and often multiple with cavity formation (Fig. 6.19) and carry a high risk of fistula formation. There is little or no inflammatory cell reaction around the larger colonies (Fig. 6.20). Morphology of the fungus is readily seen in silver preparations (Fig. 6.21) which also commonly demonstrate vessel wall invasion (Fig. 6.22).

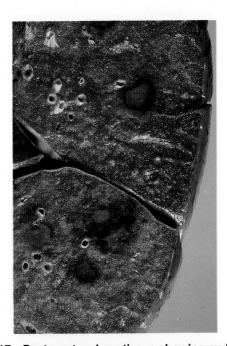

Fig. 6.17 Post mortem lung tissue showing multiple centrally pale and necrotic rounded lesions with marginal haemorrhagic appearance in a patient who died from invasive pulmonary aspergillosis.

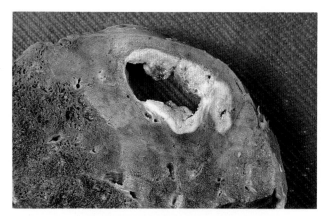

Fig. 6.18 A subpleural cavity with a necrotic lining caused by *Aspergillus fumigatus infection*. These commonly rupture into the pleura with fistula formation.

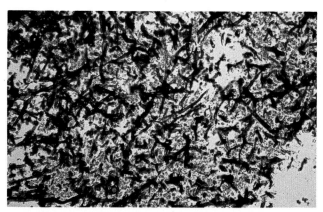

Fig. 6.21 Silver stains of *Aspergillus fumigatus* in alveoli (GMS) which demonstrates the morphology of the colonies.

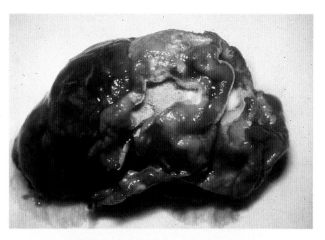

Fig. 6.19 Post mortem appearance of multiple cavities of aspergillomata (fungus balls) in lung of patient who died from acute myeloid leukaemia complicated by pulmonary aspergillosis.

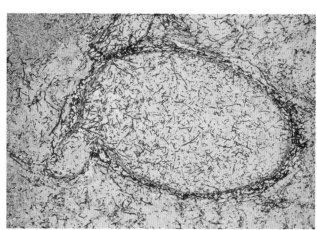

Fig. 6.22 Silver stains demonstrate the propensity of the organisms to invade blood vessel walls with luminal occlusion and infarct formation causing secondary cavitation.

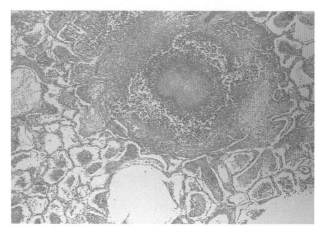

Fig. 6.20 Invasive aspergillosis: lesion of lung containing an *Aspergillus* colony. (Haematoxylin and eosin.)

CANDIDA INFECTIONS

Candida albicans is the most important yeast-like fungus to produce human disease. It is present as part of the normal flora of the mouth and gastro-intestinal tract where it is usually present in low numbers. However, in response to broad-spectrum antibiotics, poor oral hygiene and altered nutrition, overgrowth may result and produce mucosal candidosis. In severely immunocompromised patients, such as those with advanced HIV infection or profound neutropenia, severe invasive *Candida* mucositis of the mouth and oesophagus can occur and on occasions may also involve the lungs to produce a severe form of pneumonia. Pulmonary candidosis may also complicate disseminated

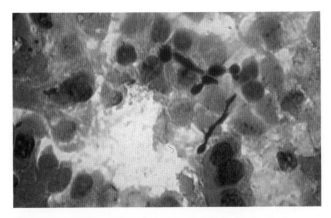

Fig. 6.23 Post mortem lung smear in a premature infant who developed disseminated candidiasis. Note presence of yeasts with pseudo-hyphal forms.

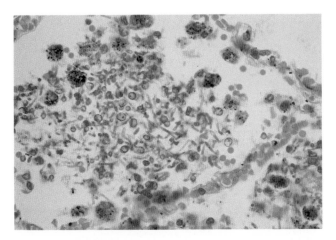

Fig. 6.24 Mycelial and yeast forms of *Candida albicans* are present in the alveoli.

Candida infection which is an increasing clinical problem, usually secondary to infected indwelling vascular lines, especially if used for intravenous feeding.

There are no pathognomic clinical features of *Candida* pneumonia. The condition is one of a spectrum of disorders that produces a non-specific infiltrate. The diagnosis requires clinical suspicion in those at risk and early resort to bronchoscopic sampling, including bronchial lavage. Treatment with amphotericin B, with or without flucytosine, remains the treatment of choice, although new azoles such as fluconazole and itraconazole are proving effective alternatives. Sadly, the diagnosis of pulmonary candidosis is often made at post mortem. Figure 6.23 shows the typical appearance of hyphal formation of *Candida* present in a post mortem lung smear, while the histopathological features of alveo-

lar filling with yeast and mycelial forms of *Candida* with associated fragmented macrophages but no cellular inflammatory reaction are demonstrated in Fig. 6.24.

CRYPTOCOCCUS NEOFORMANS PNEUMONIA

Cryptococcus neoformans is an uncommon cause of pneumonia. However, with the steady increase in the number of HIV-infected persons and the growing population of severely immunosuppressed patients, this infection is being increasingly recognized. *Cryptococcus neoformans* is a yeast-like fungus that reproduces by budding. It exists in saprophytic form within the environment, and is also found in pigeon droppings. Infection is acquired by inhalation. The lung infection is the major route for haematogenous dissemination to other sites, especially the central nervous system. Cryptococcal meningitis is the most common manifestation of this infection.

Unlike some mycoses, cryptococcosis is not restricted geographically. Although most reports in the literature have been from North America the condition is recognized worldwide. Before the HIV pandemic those at risk of invasive cryptococcosis included those with advanced malignant disease, particularly lymphoma and chronic lymphocytic leukaemia, together with those on immunosuppressive therapy, especially high dose corticosteroids. With the advent of HIV disease *Cryptococcus neoformans* has assumed greater prominence, particularly as a cause of meningitis.

Primary pulmonary infection, although uncommon, is increasingly recognized. Within the lung it may give rise to diffuse interstitial pneumonitis, a granulomatous pneumonia, and even isolated peripheral granulomata.

The clinical features of pulmonary cryptococcosis are non-specific. The presentation is often subacute and symptoms scanty. Cough is generally unproductive and pain absent unless the pleura is involved. Fever is low grade although with more advanced disease sweating, progressive shortness of breath and malaise become more prominent. The lower lobes are more commonly affected. Pleural exudate may occur. The radiographic changes are non-specific and indistinguishable from other causes of diffuse interstitial pneumonia. Examination of sputum or bronchoalveolar lavage material is usually positive for *Cryptococcus neoformans*, which grows well on both blood agar and yeast media (Fig. 6.25). A typical chest radiographic appearance is shown in

65

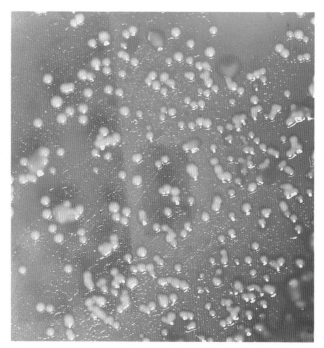

Fig. 6.25 Colonial appearance at 48 hours of *Cryptococcus neoformans* growing on selective agar. The fungus was isolated from bronchoalveolar lavage material obtained from the patient described in Fig. 6.26.

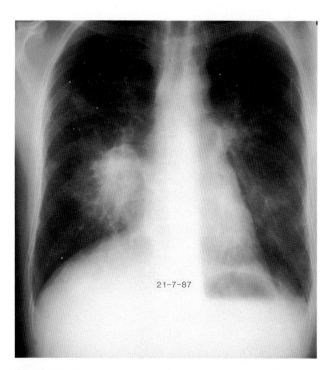

21-7-87

Fig. 6.26 Chest radiographic appearance of pulmonary cryptococcosis in a patient with AIDS. The infection is bilateral and was established by bronchoalveolar lavage and culture. Cryptococcal antigen was present in the blood. There was a satisfactory response to parenteral amphotericin B with maintenance oral fluconazole.

Fig. 6.26. The diagnosis may also be confirmed by the demonstration of circulating cryptococcal antigen using a commercial latex coagglutination method. It is important to remember that in the HIV-infected patient *Cryptococcus neoformans* may coexist with other pathogens such as *Pneumocystis carinii*.

A fatal outcome is not uncommon, especially if the diagnosis is delayed. Figure 6.27 shows multiple granulomas due to *Cryptococcus neoformans*. Diagnosis requires demonstration of the organisms, usually with the help of silver stains (Fig. 6.28).

Cryptococcus neoformans is susceptible to treatment with amphotericin B, flucytosine or fluconazole. At present amphotericin B, either alone or in combination with flucytosine, is preferred. Treatment for 4–6 weeks is usually adequate to produce cure, although

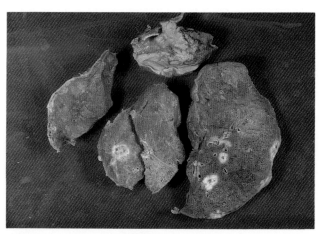

Fig. 6.27 Multiple lung granulomas due to *Cryptococcus neoformans*. Gross features are by no means specific.

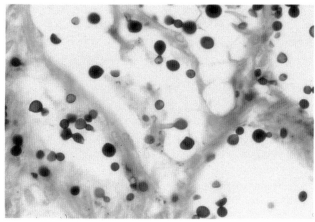

Fig. 6.28 Section of lung showing budding yeast forms of *Cryptococcus neoformans* in alveoli. Note lack of inflammatory response. This was an opportunistic infection in a renal transplant patient.

in the HIV-infected more prolonged treatment may be necessary. Fluconazole provides a useful alternative. In the HIV-infected patient long-term maintenance treatment with low dose fluconazole is necessary.

MUCORMYCOSIS

Mucormycosis is an uncommon cause of lung infection and may be due to one of several different fungi which include *Rhizopus*, *Absidia* and *Mucor* species. These are saprophytic fungi which are widely distributed in nature. Spore formation allows inhalation or direct inoculation into ulcerated skin and mucosal surfaces. Mucormycosis is largely confined to patients with haematological malignancies, those with prolonged neutropenia and also patients with diabetes mellitus.

Mucormycosis can affect the lungs, skin, gut and central nervous system although the most common manifestation is the rhinocerebral form. Here the infection is locally invasive with pain, orbital oedema and progressive loss of extraocular muscular function. Thrombosis of local vessels due to hyphal invasion of blood vessels and sinuses can result in loss of vision. Direct invasion of the underlying cranium may follow. Not surprisingly this form of mucormycosis is often fatal, although successful treatment has been reported with amphotericin B, with or without surgical debridement, and usually coincides with recover of the neutropenic state.

Pulmonary mucormycosis again largely affects the severely immunocompromised and neutropenic patient. The clinical features are non-specific but

include fever, cough and haemoptysis. The chest radiograph may show localized infiltration, often with cavitation and subsequent spread to adjacent segments. The diagnosis is made by examination of sputum or lavage material and, if possible, biopsy, although the risk of haemorrhage in many of these patients precludes this investigation. Regrettably the infection is often diagnosed at post mortem when the characteristic strap-like broad hyphae (Fig. 6.29) are seen, while in Fig. 6.30 the tendency to occur in and around blood vessels is well demonstrated.

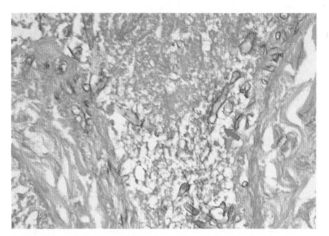

Fig. 6.30   Invasive hyphae of *Mucor* passing through pulmonary vessel wall into lumen (arrow); a common feature of this infection.

CYTOMEGALOVIRUS INFECTION

Cytomegalovirus (CMV) is one of the herpes viruses. Primary infection occurs in early life and is often asymptomatic. This is followed by a state of latency in which there is no active viral replication although subsequent reactivation in later life may produce symptomatic illness. Human disease caused by CMV is very much determined by the state of host defences. Where these are suppressed reactivation of disease is common, especially among organ transplant recipients, the HIV-infected, and patients receiving high dose immunosuppressive therapy. The lungs are involved as part of a disseminated infection in which multi-organ disease is apparent.

A common clinical presentation is in the bone marrow transplant recipient, who several weeks after successful transplantation develops progressive fever, accompanied by malaise, sweats, abnormal liver function, perhaps neutropenia and evidence of progressive pneumonitis with a minimally productive cough. Conventional bacteriological samples are

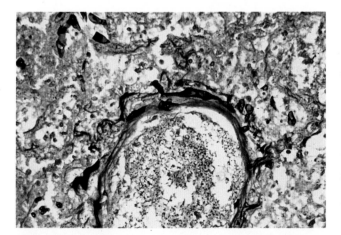

Fig. 6.29   Mucormycosis: pulmonary vessel invaded by *Mucor* hyphae which are of typical broad strap-like appearance (GMS).

unhelpful and early bronchoscope sampling, including BAL, is recommended. Cytological examination may show characteristic changes in pneumocytes as in Fig. 6.31. Further support for the diagnosis is through the detection of a positive DEAFF test as seen in Fig. 6.33. It is important to remember that CMV infection often coexists with other infectious problems. CMV disease often improves with a

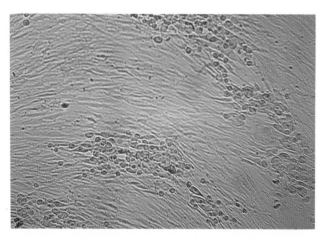

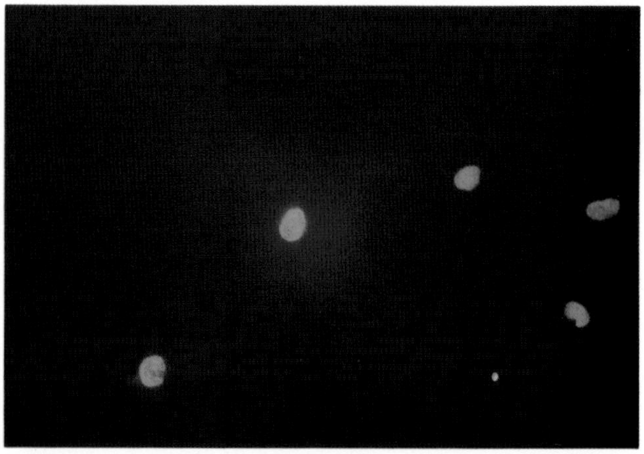

Fig. 6.31 Cytopathic effect of cytomegalovirus of MRC tissue culture cells.

Fig. 6.33 Detection of CMV in tissue culture by the DEAFF (detection of early antigen in fluorescent foci) test.

obtained by virus isolation in tissue culture but this is relatively slow. This process can be abbreviated by the use of the DEAFF test (detection of early antigen foci of fluorescence) using a specific antibody conjugate. The virus may also be demonstrated by culture or cytology in urine and may be cultured from circulating white cells. Figure 6.32 shows the typical histopathological features with the 'owl's eye' inclusion body which characterizes CMV infection. The laboratory diagnosis can be supported most rapidly

reduction in the level of immunosuppression. However, in severe cases antiviral chemotherapy is justified. At present ganciclovir or foscarnate should be considered although both carry the risk of serious toxicity, including bone marrow suppression.

STRONGYLOIDES INFECTION

An uncommon but life-threatening infection in the severely immunocompromised is that of hyperinfection with *Strongyloides stercoralis*. This ubiquitous helminth can persist in parasitic form in the gut for many years. The adult female worm produces ova which are eliminated by defaecation. In addition, infective larval forms are found in the faeces and poor personal hygiene can therefore result in autoinfection to maintain the life cycle. In the severely immunocompromised patient, especially transplant recipients, the immunological mechanisms which keep the infection in check fail and a state of hyperinfection can occur. This is associated with massive larval invasion of the tissues. The larvae penetrate the gut mucosa and migrate throughout the body, including the lungs, to produce areas of pneumonitis. The transmural larval migration through the bowel is often accompanied by bacteraemia with a mixture of organisms, while involvement of the lung can result in expectoration of larvae visible on sputum microscopy. There are no specific

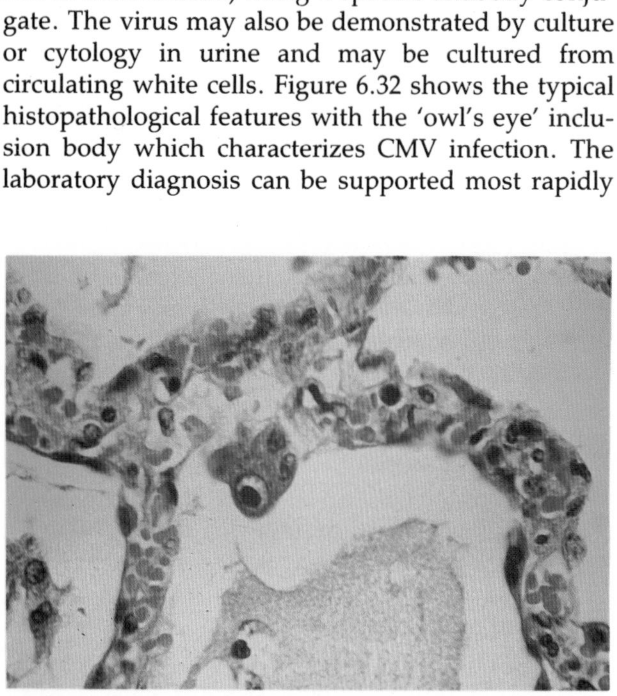

Fig. 6.32 Post mortem specimen of lung in renal transplant recipient who developed cytomegalovirus pneumonia. Note typical 'owl's eye' inclusion body within a pneumocyte nucleus which is much increased in size.

radiological features but diffuse shadowing is common. Eosinophilia may be absent. High dose thiabendazole may improve the situation but fatalities still occur. Figure 6.34 shows the typical mor-

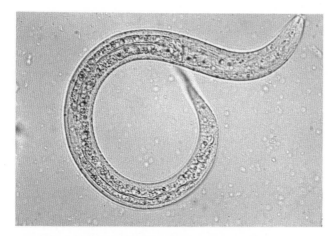

Fig. 6.34 Larva of *Strongyloides stercoralis*. This may occasionally cause a hyperinfection syndrome in severely immunosuppressed patients. Larvae migrate from the bowel to involve many tissues and may be coughed up in sputum. The infection sometimes responds to high dose thiabendazole.

phology of the filariform larva of *Strongyloides stercoralis* which has been hatched in the laboratory from ova present in the faeces.

MYCOBACTERIAL DISEASE

Patients with HIV disease are at increased risk from mycobacterial infection. This often reflects reactivation of past exposure and occurs as cell-mediated immunity wanes. These patients are also at risk from acquired mcyobacterial disease which may be caused by both *Mycobacterium tuberculosis* and also atypical mycobacteria. Infections with *M. tuberculosis* tend to occur earlier in the course of the disease and are discussed in Chapter 11. Infections with *Mycobacterium avium* complex (MAC) are increasingly recognized and often present late in the course of HIV infection. Other atypical mycobacteria are also seen from time to time. This patient population is important because of the need to diagnose and manage their mycobacterial disease, but in addition they are an important source for disseminating mycobacterial disease among other HIV-infected and non-infected persons.

In non-tuberculous mycobacterial disease bacteraemia is common and hence multi-organ involve-ment frequently occurs, often with little host response. Infection may go unrecognised for many months, and indeed often coexists with other infections such as *Pneumocystis carinii* pneumonia. Clinical features include fever, night sweats, fatigue and weight loss. There may be abdominal symptoms, including diarrhoea, while hepatosplenomegaly and lymphadenopathy are not uncommon. The diagnosis should be strongly suspected in advanced HIV disease when it may be diagnosed on the basis of a positive blood culture, positive bronchoalveolar fluid or biopsy material. Figure 6.35 demonstrates MAC in a lymph node biopsy.

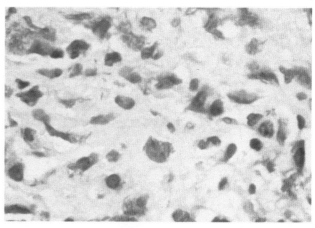

Fig. 6.35 Lymph node biopsy from a patient with AIDS who complained of fever, sweats, fatigue and weight loss. In the centre of the field is a macrophage laden with acid/alcohol-fast bacilli on Ziehl-Neelsen staining. This biopsy subsequently yielded *Mycobacterium avium-intracellulare* on culture.

KAPOSI'S SARCOMA

Kaposi's sarcoma (KS) was uncommon before the HIV pandemic when it was largely associated with low grade skin disease in the elderly. KS is now the commonest malignant manifestation of HIV disease and, with *Pneumocystis carinii* pneumonia, is now assuming the role as the leading cause of death in those with AIDS. KS may affect several body sites and in those with HIV is rarely limited to one particular area. The mouth and face are common sites. Visceral involvement is also fairly common and may remain clinically silent, unlike pulmonary KS, which has a relatively poor prognosis. Symptoms include dyspnoea, a relatively unproductive cough and occasionally fever. The chest radiograph may show a variety of features which vary from a nodular pattern to diffuse infiltration and pleural

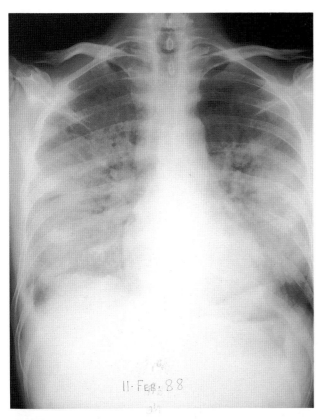

Fig. 6.36 Chest radiographic appearance of pulmonary Kaposi's sarcoma in patient with AIDS.

The diagnosis is made by bronchoscopy, which visualizes the lesions. Biopsy is hazardous because of the risk of haemorrhage. There is usually coexistent skin involvement which provides supportive evidence for the diagnosis.

To date there is little in the way of effective treatment although radiotherapy, various cytotoxic regimens and interferon have been used. For progressive KS of the lung with recurrent haemoptyses, radiotherapy is preferred.

effusion which is often blood-stained. The chest radiographic appearance of a patient with AIDS and KS is shown in Fig. 6.36. In contrast to *Pneumocystis carinii* pneumonia, the gallim scan is generally negative unless a mixed disease is present.

FURTHER READING

Cairns, M. R. and Durack, D. T. (1986) Fungal pneumonia in the immunocompromised host. In *Seminars in Respiratory Infection*, vol. 1 (ed. J. R. Hoidal), pp. 166–85. Grune & Stratton, Orlando.

Caray, S. M., Belenko, M., Fazzini, E. *et al.* (1987) Pulmonary manifestations of Kaposi's sarcoma. *Chest*, **91**, 39–43.

Fanta, C. H. and Pennington, J. E. (1989) Pneumonia in the immunocompromised host. In *Respiratory Infections: Diagnosis and Management*, 2nd edn (ed. J. E. Pennington), pp. 221–40. Raven Press, New York.

Macfarlane, J. and Finch, R. G. (1985) Pneumocystis carinii pneumonia. *Thorax*, **50**, 561–70.

O'Doherty, M. J. and Bateman, N. T. (1991) Prophylaxis and treatment of Pneumocystis carinii pneumonia. *British Journal of Hospital Medicine*, **45**, 277–83.

Scowden, E. B., Schaffner, W. and Stone, W. J. (1978) Overwhelming strongyloidiasis. An unappreciated opportunistic infection. *Medicine*, **57**, 527–44.

Sugar, A. M. (1990) Agents of mucormycosis and related species. In *Principles and Practice of Infectious Diseases*, 3rd edn (eds G. L. Mandell, R. G. Douglas and J. E. Bennett), pp. 1962–72. John Wiley and Sons, New York.

7. *Aspiration and Anaerobic Pneumonias*

INTRODUCTION

Aspiration into the bronchopulmonary area can cause a number of distinct problems. Firstly, aspiration of particulate matter, foreign bodies or large volumes of inert fluid will cause obstruction of the airways. Secondly, chemical bronchitis and pneumonitis can occur following aspiration of toxic substances, gastric acid or other substances such as lipids. Thirdly, infection is very common, usually caused by oropharyngeal bacteria. The types of bacteria will vary in different clinical circumstances and this knowledge is important when managing aspiration pneumonia.

Oropharyngeal bacteria in the previously healthy individual or person in the community will be a mixture an anaerobic bacteria, including peptostreptococci, fusobacteria and *Bacteroides* spp. Lung infection can cause necrotizing pneumonia and lung abscess. The majority of these bacteria will be sensitive to penicillin although there is an increasing problem with penicillin-resistant *Bacteroides*. In persons with poor dental hygiene or frank gingival infection, other organisms such as *Actinomycosis israelii* and *Arachnia* spp. may be encountered.

In contrast, in the patient who is severely debilitated, has had multiple prior antibiotics or has been in hospital for some while, the oropharynx will commonly have become colonized with pathogenic Gram-negative bacillary organisms such as *Proteus* spp., *Klebsiella* spp. and *Pseudomonas aeruginosa*. This will require a different management approach using combinations of such antibiotics as third generation cephalosporins, ureidopenicillins (e.g. azlocillin or ticarcillin) and quinolones (e.g. ciprofloxacin).

Illustrative case histories are given below.

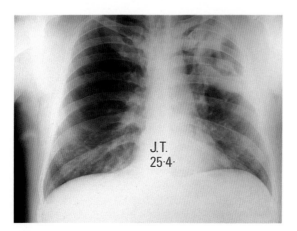

Fig. 7.1 A 30-year-old epileptic man started coughing up foul-smelling sputum 10 days after a grand mal fit. Mixed anaerobes were identified from a percutaneous lung aspirate.

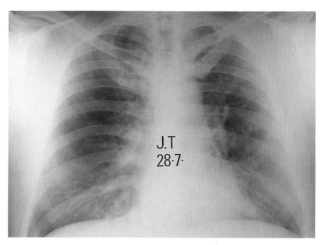

Fig. 7.2 He was treated with oral clindamycin for one month and the anaerobic aspiration abscess completely resolved. A bronchoscopy had shown no evidence of endobronchial foreign body.

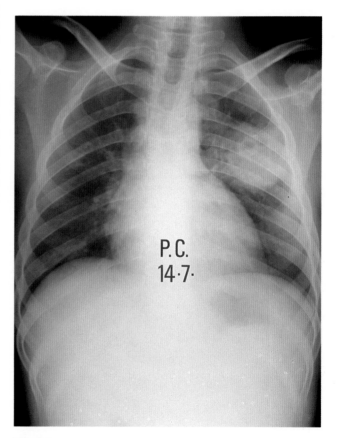

Fig. 7.3 A similar problem was encountered with a mentally retarded 40-year-old man with a left upper lobe lung abscess. Some aspirated food debris was removed from the left upper lobe bronchus at bronchoscopy and mixed penicillin-sensitive anaerobes cultured from a percutaneous needle aspiration. He made a good recovery with a prolonged course of oral amoxycillin.

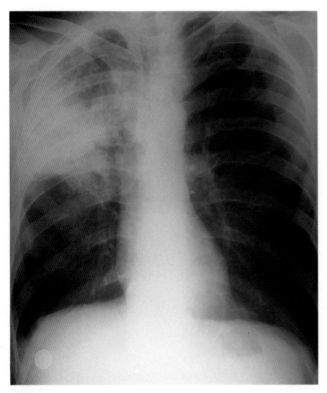

Fig. 7.4 A 40-year-old alcoholic presented with a severe right upper lobe pneumonia. Gram stain of pus aspirated at bronchoscopy showed large numbers of neutrophils together with Gram-positive cocci. In spite of not having received any prior antibiotics, no pathogens were cultured on aerobic culture plates, suggesting a diagnosis of anaerobic infection. He recovered with a prolonged course of parenteral penicillin although some cavitation developed in the right upper lobe.

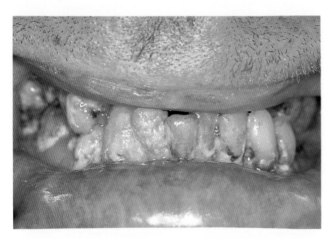

Fig. 7.5 In his case gross dental caries almost certainly contributed to his anaerobic pulmonary infection.

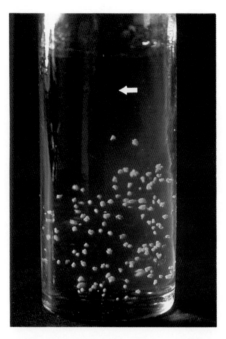

Fig. 7.6 *Streptococcus milleri* growing on nutrient agar. Note absence of colonies near surface (arrow). *Stretococcus milleri* is associated with a variety of suppurative infections, including necrotizing pneumonia, lung abscesses, empyema and intra-abdominal abscesses, particularly of the liver. It is a microaerophilic organism, which produces a characteristic growth pattern in nutrient broth with absence of colonies near the oxygen-richer surface.

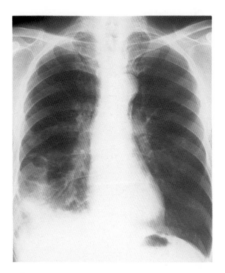

Fig. 7.7 *Streptococcus milleri* was isolated from bronchial aspirates from the right lower lobe of a man with acute pneumonia. He presented six months later with a left upper lobe pneumonia and a diagnosis of achalasia of the cardia was made which had resulted in aspiration and recurrent anaerobic pneumonia. Surgical correction of his achalasia resulted in no further episodes of pneumonia.

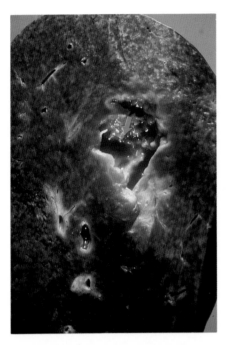

Fig. 7.8 The *Streptococcus milleri* illustrated in Fig. 7.6 was isolated from blood and pleural fluid cultures of a patient with a right empyema who failed to respond despite high dose penicillin. An associated liver abscess was found at autopsy (arrow).

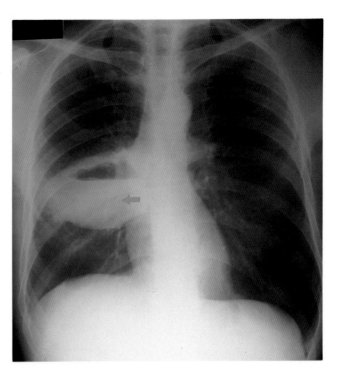

Fig. 7.10 A lung abscess with fluid level (arrow) is seen in the apex of the right lower lobe of a 65-year-old male cigarette smoker.

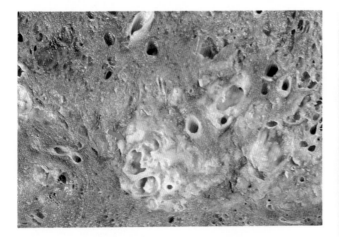

Fig. 7.9 The lung showed focal suppuration (arrow).

Fig. 7.11 A CT scan of the chest confirms a smooth-walled abscess with a fluid level but there is also a small mass obstructing the draining bronchus (arrow). The anaerobic abscess resolved with penicillin therapy and a small endobronchial squamous cell carcinoma was subsequently resected by lobectomy.

ANAEROBIC INFECTION SECONDARY TO BRONCHIAL OBSTRUCTION

A cavitating and necrotic squamous cell carcinoma can sometimes mimic a primary lung abscess but a thicker irregular wall is more suggestive of tumour (Fig. 7.12).

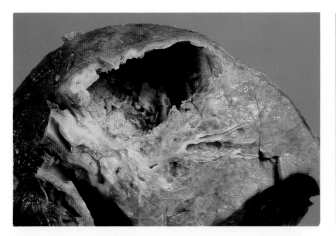

Fig. 7.12   Cavitating squamous cell lung cancer that can mimic a lung abscess, although in this case the thick wall is more suggestive of a tumour.

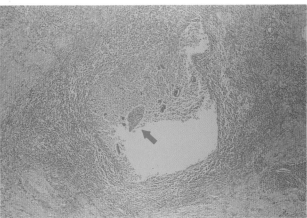

Fig. 7.14   A low power view of part of the resected 'mass' revealed a bronchus nearly obstructed by inflammatory granulation tissue with a mass of colonies of *actinomyces* in the lumen (arrow).

ASPIRATION PNEUMONIA DUE TO *ACTINOMYCES* AND *ARACHNIA*

Actinomyces and *Arachnia* species are constituents of the normal flora of plaque, carious teeth, periodontal clefts and tonsillar crypts. Pleuropulmonary infection follows aspiration of infected oral debris and is characterized by a chronic suppurative and invasive process unimpeded by traditional anatomical barriers.

Most commonly the clinical picture mimics tuberculosis or lung cancer with an enlarging lesion on the chest radiograph and constitutional symptoms. Diagnosis is difficult and is sometimes made only after lung biopsy or surgical resection.

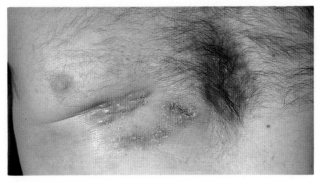

Fig. 7.15   A 40-year-old man presented with a month's history of fevers, weight loss, right chest pain and dry cough. Multiple pustules and skin induration were present over the right anterior chest wall and *Actinomyces israelii* and *Actinobacillus actinomycetem comitans* were cultured from the pus.

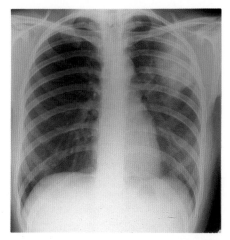

Fig. 7.13   A 45-year-old female cigarette smoker presented with a two-month history of weight loss, cough and malaise and an enlarging shadow on her chest radiograph which required resection to make a diagnosis.

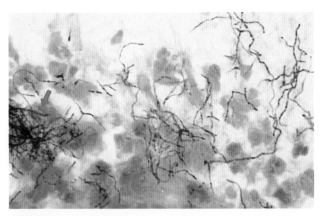

Fig. 7.16   Gram stain of the pus from the discharging sinus is illustrated. Note the typical fine branching morphology of *Actinomyces israelii*. The 'sulphur granules' colonies are just visible in the exudate (arrow).

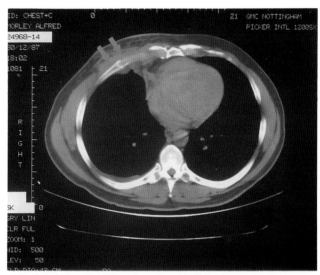

Fig. 7.19 The corresponding CT scan slice shows pleural shadowing (single arrow) with evidence of extension of the infection into subcutaneous tissue of the right anterior chest (double arrows). Reproduced by permission of Baillière Tindall.

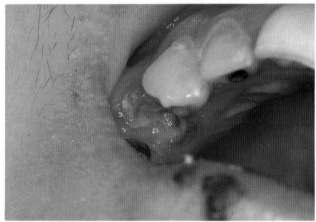

Fig. 7.20 An infected tooth socket was the possible source of infection. Healing herpes labialis is seen on the lower lip. He made a complete recovery following prolonged penicillin therapy.

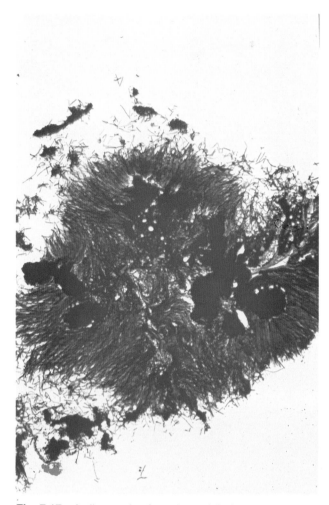

Fig. 7.17 A silver stain of a colony of *Actinomyces* demonstrating the structure of a 'sulphur granule' as a dense collection of filamentous organisms.

NON-INFECTIVE LIPOID ASPIRATION PNEUMONIA

There are two forms of lipoid pneumonia. Exogenous lipid material may be aspirated from the pharynx or oesophagus. Examples include liquid paraffin formerly used as a laxative, accidental inhalation of oil droplets during explosions or fires or aspiration of enteral liquid feeds following incorrect intratracheal placement of nasogastric feeding tubes or where there is oesophageal obstruction.

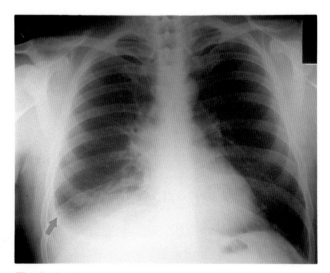

Fig. 7.18 His chest radiograph showed pulmonary and pleural shadowing in the right lower zone (arrow). Reproduced by permission of Baillière Tindall.

Endogenous lipoid pneumonia involves the accumulation of locally generated lipid material distal to bronchial obstruction, particularly from bronchial carcinoma.

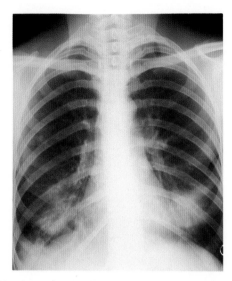

Fig. 7.21 An example of exogenous lipoid pneumonia is shown by a 69-year-old spinster who had swallowed liquid paraffin daily for a number of years. Bilateral basal patchy shadowing was present and fat-laden macrophages were found in her sputum. The chest radiograph gradually cleared on stopping liquid paraffin. Reproduced by permission of Baillière Tindall.

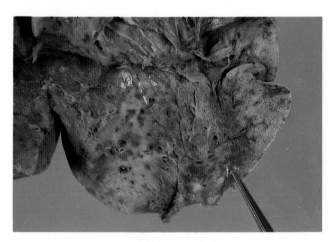

Fig. 7.22 In this fatal case of exogenous lipoid pneumonia, due to achalasia of the cardia, yellow fatty foci of consolidated lung are seen (arrow) caused by large numbers of foamy macrophages containing large amounts of lipid.

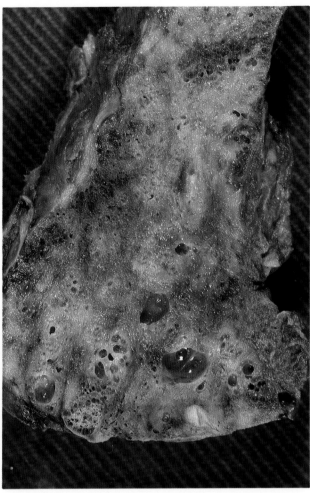

Fig. 7.23 A patient with achalasia of the cardia died of pneumonia. Examination of the lung revealed multiple oil-filled cavities or 'paraffinomas', with associated fibrotic reaction in the lung caused by chronic aspiration of liquid paraffin taken to ease swallowing. Note the shiny oily appearance of material in the larger spaces.

FURTHER READING

Finegold, S. M. (1989) Aspiration pneumonia lung abscess and empyema. In *Respiratory Infections: Diagnosis and Management* 2nd edn (ed. J. E. Pennington) pp. 264–75. Raven Press, New York.

Johanson, W. G. and Harris, G. D. (1980) Aspiration pneumonia, anaerobic infections and lung abscess. *Medical Clinics of North America*, **64**, 385–94.

Kinnear, W. J. M. and Macfarlane, J. T. (1990) A survey of thoracic actinomycosis. *Respiratory Medicine*, **84**, 57–9.

8. Uncommon or Geographically Restricted Respiratory Tract Infections

INTRODUCTION

In this chapter we include a pot pourri of conditions that do not easily fit into other chapters but which offer an additional perspective on the range of conditions affecting the lung. Many of these conditions are either rare or only seen when imported into the UK/Western Europe. Many are geographically restricted to the tropics and subtropics while the mycoses are all seen in the Americas. Paragonimiasis is also found to a large extent in the Far East and Indian subcontinent. The material available to us has been limited and therefore does not carry the claim to be comprehensive. Included in this section are examples of bacterial, fungal, protozoal and helminthic disorders.

BRUCELLOSIS

Brucellosis is an important health problem worldwide, as well as resulting in serious economic losses in dairy herds. There are several species of brucellae, of which *Brucella abortus*, *B. melitensis* and *B. suis* are the best known; these affect cattle, goats and pigs respectively. Direct contact with infected tissues or ingestion of contaminated meat, and particularly dairy products, is the usual route of acquisition, although inhalation of infectious aerosols is also recognized. In parts of the Middle East and Eastern Mediterranean it is extremely common. Brucellosis presents acutely following an incubation of 2–3 weeks, with fever, sweating, rigors, malaise, headaches and often myalgia and arthralgia. The lymph nodes may be palpable and the spleen enlarged. A variety of complications can arise. This includes bone and articular infection, meningo-encephalitis, epididymo-orchitis and occasionally skin eruptions. The lung may be involved by inhalation or bacteria spread. Cough is not unusual in acute brucellosis and abnormalities of the chest radiograph may be present in approximately one fifth of patients, including enlarged hilar lymph nodes, miliary shadowing, pleural effusion, lung abscess, localized areas of infiltration and nodular lesions. Figure 8.1 illustrates lung involvement with bacteraemic *B. melitensis* infection. The diagnosis is usually made on the basis of positive blood cultures which should be incubated for up to six weeks in an atmosphere enriched with carbon dioxide. Serological support for the diagnosis can be made with paired sera demonstrating a rise in antibodies. Acute brucellosis usually responds to a combination of doxycycline 200 mg/day and rifampicin 600–900 mg/ day for six weeks.

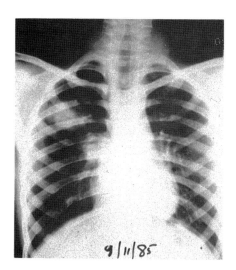

Fig. 8.1   Right upper lobe granulomatous shadowing with hilar lymphadenopathy in an 11-year-old Kuwaiti boy with bacteraemic *Brucella melitensis* infection.

FUNGAL INFECTIONS

A number of fungal diseases are geographically restricted. Among these, the dimorphic fungi responsible for histoplasmosis, blastomycosis, coccidioidomycosis and paracoccidioidomycosis present an interesting spectrum of disease in which the lung may or may not be the primary target.

Histoplasmosis

In the case of histoplasmosis, caused by *Histoplasma capsulatum*, the host response to infection is a major determinant of the pattern of disease which has similarities to turberculosis with regard to the sequence of events. Primary infection often goes unnoticed and reactivated disease, although affecting a minority of those infected, presents a more serious health problem. Primary infection may cause an acute hypersensitivity pneumonitis which can produce significant disease and be a source of diagnostic confusion in the absence of a positive geographic history. The disease is largely seen in the United States, in areas adjacent to the Ohio and Mississippi rivers, where the spores are widely distributed in the soil. Inhalation of spores produces delayed hypersensitivity with skin test conversion to histoplasmin.

Symptoms may develop about two weeks after exposure and vary in severity. They include fever, myalgia, headache and fatigue and occasionally gastrointestinal symptoms. Shortness of breath can be profound with heavy exposure. Radiographic changes are common with diffuse infiltration and hilar lymph node enlargement.

Acute disease is usually self-limiting but occasionally may require a short course of amphotericin B for its control. More serious is the subsequent reactivational form of the disease which can effect many organs, including the lungs. Figure 8.2 provides an example of disseminated disease. The HIV pandemic has seen an increase in disseminated histoplasmosis and should be considered in those geographically exposed. The fungus may be isolated in biopsy material from reactivated disease, but is rarely detected in primary infections. Figure 8.3 shows the typical cultural features.

Histoplasma capsulatum var *duboisii* is a variant of *H.*

capsulatum and is prevalent in Africa, where it produces a different spectrum of disease. Focal lesions are largely confined to the skin and bones and rarely affect the lungs. Figure 8.4 is an example of cutaneous involvement which produces wart-like papular lesions. Amphotericin B is highly effective.

The histopathology of the more common 'inactive' granulomatous primary infection shows features somewhat similar to an old primary tuberculosis focus with a discrete centrally fibrotic lesion and marginal mononuclear and lymphoid inflammatory cell infiltrate (Fig. 8.5). Even in very old lesions it is usually possible to find histiocytic cell clusters with a foamy cytoplasm (Fig. 8.6) in which organisms can be demonstrated by Giemsa or silver stains.

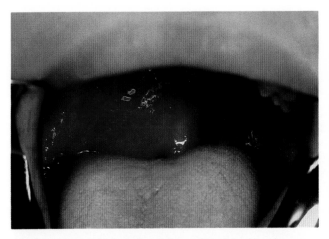

Fig. 8.2 Histoplasmosis of the soft palate. Tumour was suspected but the diagnosis was made by biopsy which demonstrated the presence of histoplasmosis. Complete recovery occurred with a course of intravenous amphotericin B.

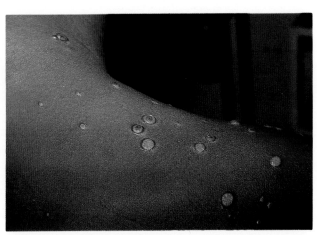

Fig. 8.4 Skin lesions of *Histoplasma duboisii* on the shoulder of a Nigerian man.

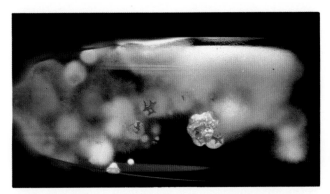

Fig. 8.3 *Histoplasma capsulatum* on mould agar after 24 days incubation at 30°C. The fungus was isolated from the urine of a patient with AIDS who was suffering from disseminated histoplasmosis. He came from near Columbus, Ohio.

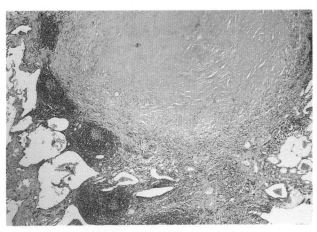

Fig. 8.5 Low power view of inactive *Histoplasma capsulatum* granuloma in lung.

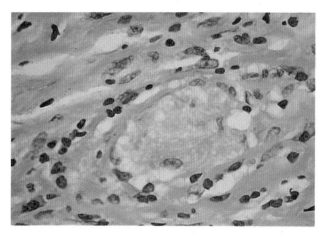

Fig. 8.6   A small collection of histiocytes in the wall of the pulmonary lesion seen in Fig. 8.5. Note 'foamy' appearance of cytoplasm. Organisms can be demonstrated as in Fig. 8.8 with Giemsa or silver stains.

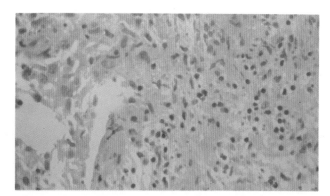

Fig. 8.7   Haematoxylin and eosin stained section of a reactivated histoplasma focus showing a characteristic foamy appearance.

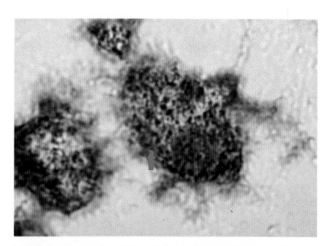

Fig. 8.8   Gomori methenamine silver stained section of a more active *Histoplasma* infection showing the intracellular organisms with surrounding clear capsular zones (arrow).

In the more active or reactivated lesions, numerous organisms can be seen on haematoxylin and eosin preparations with the characteristic clear zone (Fig. 8.7) and the numerous intracytoplasmic encapsulated yeast forms are easily demonstrated in a silver stain (Fig. 8.8).

Blastomycosis

Blastomycosis is caused by *Blastomyces dermatitidis*. The infection is prevalent throughout the Mid-West of the United States. Although acquired through inhalation of spores, haematogenous spread involves the skin, bones, genitourinary tract and lungs. Like histoplasmosis, primary infection often goes unnoticed but may produce a hypersensitivity pneumonitis. Recurrent infection produces a variety of features according to the target site. The diagnosis must be confirmed by bronchial lavage examination (Fig. 8.9) or biopsy examination, which reveals the typical yeast forms within the tissues. Culture of biopsy material produces the typical colonial appearance on yeast agar (Fig. 8.10). Ketoconazole is the preferred agent to treat blastomycosis; amphotericin B is reserved for those intolerant or unresponsive to ketoconazole or where CNS disease is present.

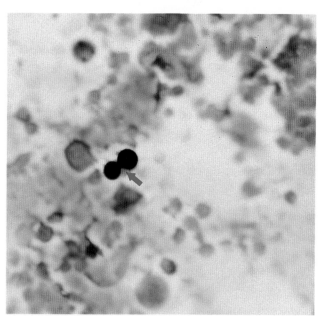

Fig. 8.9   This shows a cytological preparation stained by Gomori's methenamine silver from a bronchial aspirate sample of a case of pulmonary infection by *Blastomyces dermatitidis*. Note the broad band between these yeast-like organisms (arrow). Similar cytology samples can be an important diagnostic method for identification of severe fungal and other infections.

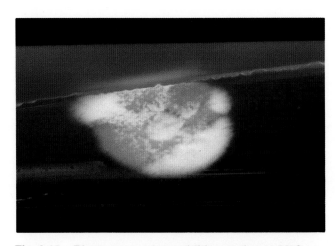

Fig. 8.10 *Blastomyces dermatiditis* growing at 30°C on mould agar and isolated from the bone marrow of a patient with extensive pulmonary blastomycosis. The patient had lived in North Carolina, USA all his life.

monly affected. The disease is uncommon in children and young adults. The primary infection is subclinical and reactivation is very much dependent upon the integrity of the host's immune system. It is not surprising, therefore, that the disease has become more common, particularly among those infected with the HIV virus. Clinical manifestations vary considerably but the lungs are often involved with widespread, usually bilateral, symmetrical infiltrates, particularly involving the basal segments. Healing is by fibrosis and may be accompanied by bullous formation. Symptoms include progressive shortness of breath, cough, occasional haemoptyses and chest discomfort. Symptoms relevant to other sites may also be present. The diagnosis is made by identification of budding *P. braziliensis* in sputum, exudate or lung biopsy material in which the histological features are pathognomonic on morphology of the organisms (Figs 8.12 and 8.13). Serological tests

Coccidioidomycosis and paracoccidioidomycosis

Other mycoses include coccidioidomycosis and paracoccidioidomycosis which are predominantly found in North and Central America respectively. Coccidioidomycosis has a natural history similar to that of tuberculosis.

Figure 8.11 illustrates the cytologial diagnosis in a bronchial aspirate. In contrast, paracoccidioidomycosis predominantly affects the skin, mucous membranes, lymphoid tissues and adrenals. It is caused by *Paracoccidioides brasiliensis*, which is thought to be acquired by inhalation. Males are much more com-

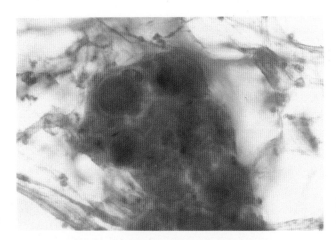

Fig. 8.11 This endosporulating spherical fungal organism (*Coccidioides immitis*) can often be demonstrated in cytological preparations when culture techniques yield negative results. PAS and/or silver stains can be used on touch preparations of the cut surface of excised lesions or on fine needle aspirates.

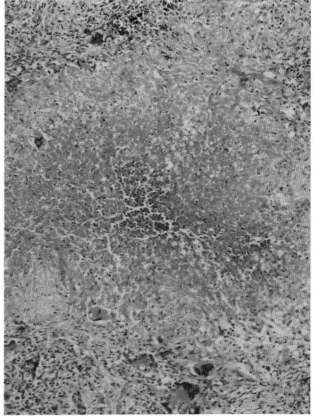

Fig. 8.12 Low power view of lung from a fatal case of paracoccidioidomycosis. There is a central necrosis with surrounding granulomatous inflammation in which large multinucleate cells containing *P. braziliensis* are prominent.

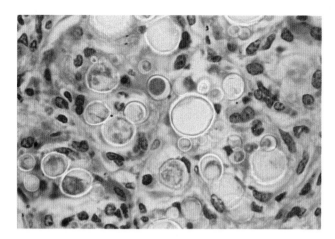

Fig. 8.13 Higher power view of *P. braziliensis* organisms in yeast-like and intracellular endosporulating spherical forms.

are helpful in both the diagnosis and assessment of response to treatment. The latter includes amphotericin B and ketoconazole, which is currently the drug of choice.

AMOEBIASIS

Amoebiasis is caused by *Entamoeba histolytica*. The disease is prevalent throughout the tropics, subtropics and other parts of the world, especially where sanitation is poor and faecal–oral transmission common. The cysts are hardy and survive in the environment for many weeks. In the UK and other developed countries infection is uncommon and is primarily related to imported disease. *Entamoeba histolytica* can also be transmitted by anal intercourse and as such is one cause of the 'Gay Bowel Syndrome .

The primary target for amoebic infection is the gut; following the ingestion of cyst forms, most persons remain asymptomatic. In those who develop symptomatic disease this ranges from non-invasive infection to the more familiar amoebic dysentery largely affecting the caecum and pelvic colon, with the potential for severe colitis, perforation and toxic megacolon. Severe disease is due to invasion of the mucosa and submucosa by trophozoites. The severity of the disease is proportional to the parasitic load. Subacute and chronic forms of colitis are recognized but uncommon, as is the development of an inflammatory mass (amoeboma) and perianal ulceration.

The ability to invade the bowel permits spread to the liver via the portal venous system where it may establish an amoebic liver abscess. These may be single or multiple and vary in size, but have the potential to spread contiguously to produce peritonitis, pericarditis, a reactive pleural effusion and amoebic abscess of the lung. The latter complication is relatively uncommon.

Figure 8.14 shows the appearance of an amoebic liver abscess on ultrasound in a patient who also had involvement of the right lung (Fig. 8.15). He presented with right upper quadrant pain and expectoration of 'anchovy sauce' sputum as a result of spontaneous rupture of the abscess into the bronchial tree (Fig. 8.16). The colour of the abscess material can range from pale cream through to red–brown and is due to the variation in blood loss into the abscess.

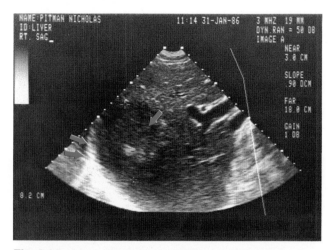

Fig. 8.14 Liver ultrasound of a 25-year-old airline steward with an amoebic liver abscess (single arrow) below diaphragms (double arrow).

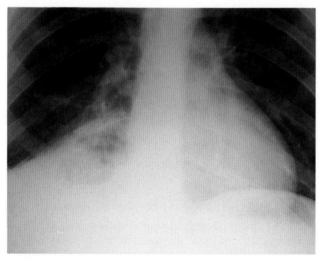

Fig. 8.15 Chest radiograph of same patient showing consolidation and collapse at right base associated with a raised diaphragm.

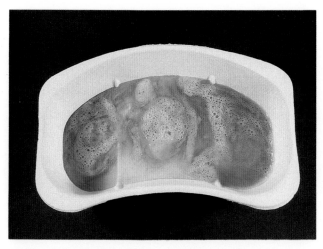

Fig. 8.16 'Anchovy sauce' coughed up when the liver abscess discharged through the diaphragm and right lower lobe (same patient as in Figs 8.14 and 8.15).

testing is also valuable in the diagnosis of invasive amoebic disease including liver abscess since the majority of patients will have an elevated antibody titre by techniques such as indirect haemagglutination. Ultrasound or CT examination are generally positive in amoebic liver abscess. Needle aspiration under ultrasound control is extremely helpful in confirming the nature of the abscess and differentiating it from the more common pyogenic liver abscess.

The treatment of choice for all forms of symptomatic amoebiasis is metronidazole for 5–10 days which is curative in the majority of patients. Emetine is now rarely used except in those intolerant of metronidazole. Cyst excretors without evidence of tissue invasion may be treated with diloxanide furoate to clear gut carriage. Advice on personal hygiene is important in order to prevent person to person spread. Improvements in sanitation offer the only real hope for more widespread control of this infection in endemic countries.

The diagnosis of amoebiasis is confirmed microbiologically and histopathologically. The parasite is present within the faeces in amoebic gut disease. In acute dysentery a fresh stool often shows motile amoebic trophozoites which typically contain ingested red blood cells. These amoebae rapidly undergo encystation on cooling and can still be identified and provide supportive diagnosis in the presence of a compatible clinical picture. Sigmoidoscopy and biopsy offer the opportunity for histopathological comfirmation. Figure 8.17 demonstrates numerous parasites on PAS staining. Serological

PARAGONIMIASIS

Paragonimiasis is one of a number of helminthic infections that may involve the lung. It is caused by the lung fluke *Paragonismus westermani*, which is particularly common throughout the Far East and Indian subcontinent, and in certain parts of Central and South America. The adult worm has a predilection for the lung bronchioles. Ova can therefore be detected in the sputum as well as the stool of infected persons. Although frequently asymptomatic, a variety of symptoms can occur and include a cough which may be productive of blood-stained sputum, while a pleural effusion, lung abscess and pleuritic chest pain and features that suggest chronic bronchitis can occur. Eosinophilia is usual. Figure 8.18 shows the typical appearance of the ova of *P. westermani* in expectorated sputum. Praziquantal is the agent of choice and is usually curative.

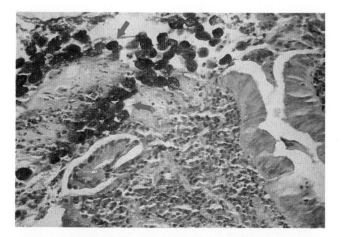

Fig. 8.17 PAS-stained section of a rectal biopsy with *Entamoeba histolytica* (arrows) infection of the rectum. The patient failed to complete a course of metronidazole and declined follow-up. Three months later he presented with an amoebic liver abscess and secondary involvement of the pleural space.

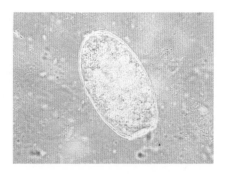

Fig. 8.18 Ova of *Paragonimus westermani* in sputum.

HYDATID DISEASE

Hydatid disease (echinococcosis) is caused by *Echinococcus granulosus*. The dog is the definitive host for the adult worm while sheep and cattle are intermediary hosts which become infected through eating contaminated dog faeces. The life cycle is completed when the dog ingests larval-infested beef or lamb. Man is secondarily infected through contact with ova from contaminated dog faeces. The ova are extremely hardy and survive many months within the environment. Following ingestion, excystation and penetration of the mesenteric blood vessel permit spread to the liver and other sites in which the hydatid cysts develop. Within the cyst is a germinal layer which gives rise to the 'brood capsule'. The cyst is filled with fluid and from the brood capsules arise the daughter cysts. Each hydatid cyst increases slowly in size and produces ill health by compression of adjacent structures.

Echinococcosis is found in cattle and sheep-producing areas of the world and is particularly common in countries adjacent to the Eastern Mediterranean. Infection is also endemic in parts of North Wales.

The disease is clinically silent for many years, although massive liver enlargement may produce a sensation of dragging or heaviness. Compression of the biliary tree can lead to obstruction or cholangitis whilst its rupture into the peritoneal cavity or pleural space produces an inflammatory reaction. Many other organs can be involved. Allergic symptoms of asthma and urticaria are uncommon although eosinophilia is usual.

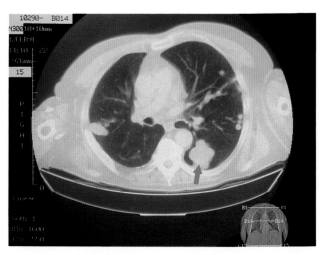

Fig. 8.20 Separate CT cuts of the thorax showed other cysts in the lung (arrow).

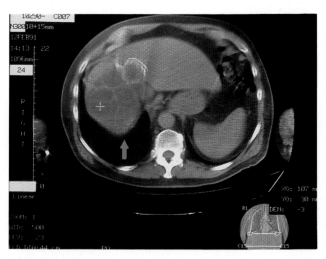

Fig. 8.21 CT scans of the abdomen showed hydatid cysts in the liver (arrow).

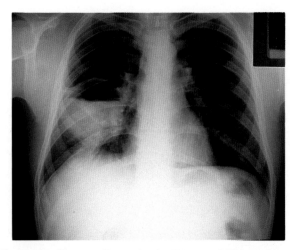

Fig. 8.19 Chest radiograph of a 55-year-old Welsh farmer with hydatid disease of the lung. He initially presented with ron-specific abdominal discomfort and was found to have an enlarged liver on clinical examination.

Surgical removal of cysts is the preferred management. Caution is essential to avoid seeding of body cavities. Albendazole may prove effective in inoperable cases and is superior to mebendazole. Figure 8.22 shows the contents of a cyst removed surgically, while Fig. 8.23 shows the appearance of a scolex within the cyst fluid. Fig. 8.24 illustrates the gross pathological appearances of a lung infected by hydatid disease while Fig. 8.25 shows the laminated membranous chitinous outer wall of a removed old cyst.

The importance of the safe disposal of infected animal carcasses, which should be kept separate from dogs, provides a means for control of this disease, although the practicalities of this approach are not so straightforward.

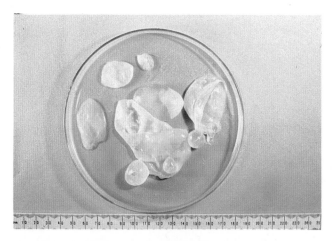

Fig. 8.22 Contents of a hydatid cyst removed at surgery from a patient with widespread abdominal disease and pleural involvement.

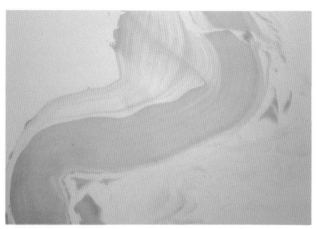

Fig. 8.25 Wall of hydatid cyst showing laminated membrane and amorphous chitinous outer cyst wall.

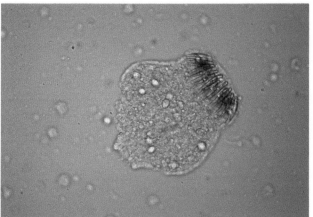

Fig. 8.23 Close-up of a hydatid scolex. Note hooklets at one end.

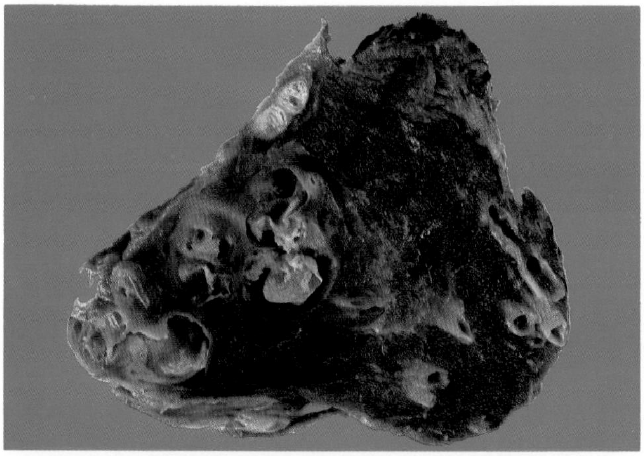

FURTHER READING

Chapman, S. W. (1990) Blastomyces dermatitiis. In *Principles and Practice of Infectious Diseases*, 3rd edn (eds G. L. Mandell, R. G. Douglas Jr and J. E. Bennett), pp. 1999–2008. John Wiley and Sons, New York.

Kubitschek, K. R., Peters, J., Nickeson, D. *et al.* (1985). Amebiasis presenting as pleuropulmonary disease. *Western Journal of Medicine*, **142**, 203–7.

Lloyd, J. E., Des Prez, R. M. and Goodwin, R. A. Jr (1990) *Histoplasma capsulatum.* In *Principles and Practice of Infectious Diseases*, 3rd edn (eds G. L. Mandell, R. G. Douglas Jr and J. E. Bennett), pp. 1989–99. John Wiley and Sons, New York.

Restrepo, A. M. (1990) *Paracoccidioides brasiliensis.* In *Principles and Practice of Infectious Diseases*, 3rd edn (eds G. L. Mandell, R. G. Douglas Jr and J. E. Bennett, pp. 2028–31. John Wiley and Sons, New York.

Stevens, D. A. (1990) *Coccidioides immitis.* In *Principles and Practice of Infectious Diseases*, 3rd edn (eds G. L. Mandell, R. G. Douglas and J. E. Bennett), pp. 2008–17. John Wiley and Sons, New York.

Taylor, D. H. and Morris, D. L. (1988) The current management of hydatid disease. *British Journal of Clinical Practice*, **42**, 401–5.

Weinberg, A. N. (1989) Unusual bacterial pneumonias including those caused by Neisseria, Branhamella, *Pseudomonas pseudomallei, Bacillus anthracis, Brucella* species, *Pasteurella multocida, Yersinia pestis* (Plague), and *Francisella tularensis.* In *Respiratory Infections: Diagnosis and Management*, 2nd edn (ed. J. E. Pennington), pp. 403–25. Raven Press, New York.

Fig. 8.24 Hydatid disease of the lung in which there are several cysts, some with clear fluid contents and others older and partly calcified.

9. Complications of Pneumonia

Complications of pneumonia can be divided into early, infective complications and delayed structural damage to the lung or bronchial tree.

EARLY INFECTIVE COMPLICATIONS

Pleural effusion and empyema

Non-infected sympathetic pleural exudates are not uncommon following any type of bacterial pneumonia. These often arise within a few days of the start of the pneumonia and will disappear gradually with the recovery of the pneumonia. It is essential to sample such pleural effusions to confirm that an empyema is not forming and to hasten resolution by drainage. Such effusions will be exudates, with high protein and some inflammatory cells but without organisms discovered on stain or culture.

A more serious complication is the development of an empyema or infected pleural fluid. The incidence of empyema varies with the cause of the pneumonia. In absolute numbers pneumococcal pneumonia is still the most common cause of empyema worldwide but probably occurs in only 1% or 2% of lobar pneumonias. In contrast empyemas develop more frequently in patients with staphylococcal, streptococcal, Gram-negative and anaerobic pneumonias probably due to increased production of local toxins that promote spread of infection and tissue necrosis.

An empyema should be suspected in anyone who is making a slow improvement following pneumonia, particularly if they remain with fevers, anorexia and pleural pain. Cough and sputum production may be absent unless a bronchopleural fistula has developed.

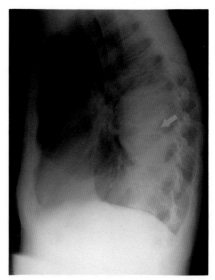

Fig. 9.2 The left lateral radiograph showed a characteristic pleural-based mass (arrow) suggestive of loculated pleural fluid.

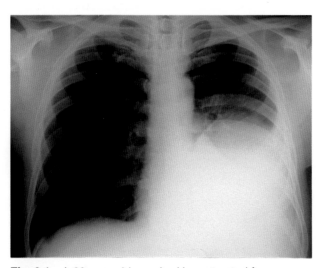

Fig. 9.1 A 60-year-old man had been treated for pneumonia by his general practitioner three weeks previously. Although he initially improved with antibiotics and his cough resolved he continued to complain of fevers, night sweats, malaise and left pleural pain. The chest radiograph showed shadowing at the left base.

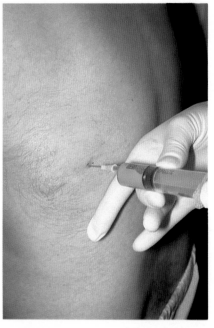

Fig. 9.3 Aspiration of the chest revealed thick pus from which *Staphylococcus aureus* was cultured. On occasions, pus may be too thick to be aspirated with an ordinary needle and this may mask the correct diagnosis.

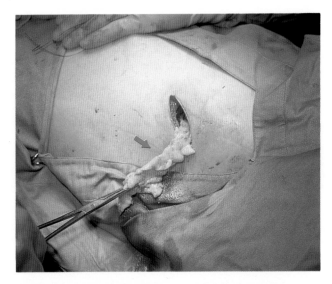

Fig. 9.6 Large sheets of fibrin and debris were also removed from the empyema cavity (arrow) prior to inserting a large bore drainage tube (Fig. 9.6). It was hardly surprising that drainage through a standard chest drain was inadequate, having seen the amount of solid debris in the empyema cavity.

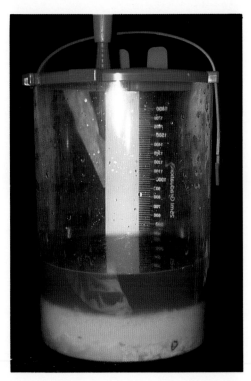

Fig. 9.4 An intercostal chest drain was inserted and 500 ml of pus was removed into the drainage bottle.

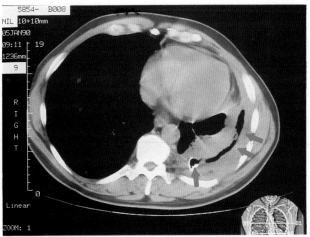

Fig. 9.7 A subsequent CT scan of the chest showed the tube (one arrow) lying within a very thick-walled empyema cavity (two arrows). There is associated loss of volume of that hemithorax. Surgical decortication was subsequently carried out successfully.

Lung abscess formation and cavitation

The bacterial pathogens that are associated with empyema formation are also more likely to cause lung necrosis and cavitation within an area of pneumonic consolidation. Such cavitation will complicate recovery and be associated with some permanent structural lung damage. Cavitation is uncommon with pneumococcal pneumonia, except with

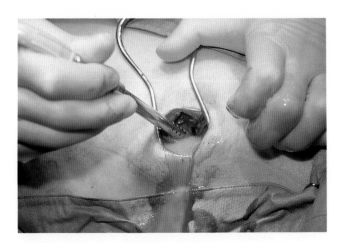

Fig. 9.5 To improve drainage a rib resection was performed and at operation further amounts of thick pus were drained.

serotype 3 infection (see Chapter 4). It is commoner with staphylococcal pneumonia, occurring in about 20%.

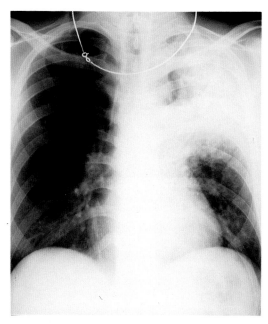

Fig. 9.8 A 22-year-old man presented with left upper lobe pneumonia following influenza virus infection. Gram-positive cocci were identified in a purulent sputum specimen from which *Staphylococcus aureus* was cultured in heavy growth. Cavitation developed and his temperature only gradually settled over one week with appropriate antibiotics. In all he was treated with four weeks of flucloxacillin, made a full clinical recovery but was left with some linear scarring in his left upper lobe.

Distant infection

Spread of infection is possible in bacteraemic pneumonia but is uncommon. Complications to consider include meningitis, endocarditis, septic arthritis and renal abscesses.

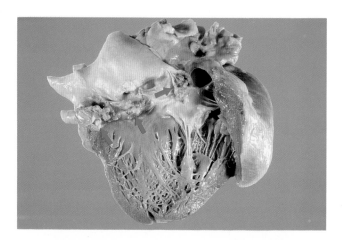

Fig. 9.10 Vegetations of acute aortic valve (arrows) were discovered at post mortem in a 30-year-old man who developed fulminating bacteraemic staphylococcal pneumonia.

LATE COMPLICATIONS

Although the lung has remarkable powers of recovery, particularly following pneumococcal pneumonia, healing with fibrosis can also occur. On a

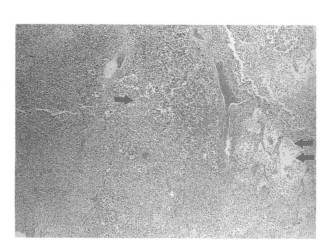

Fig. 9.9 This illustrates the lung histology of an elderly women who died of *Klebsiella* pneumonia. Abscess formation can be seen to be developing (one arrow) in an area of lobular consolidation in which some alveolar walls can still be distinguished (two arrows).

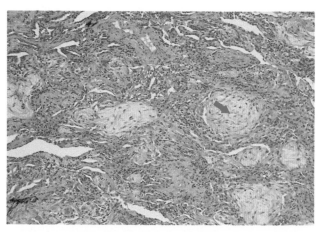

Fig. 9.11 In this example of organizing pneumonia, the alveolar exudate instead of resolving is being organized with production of fibrosis and obliteration of alveolar spaces (arrow).

macroscopic scale this can result in areas of organizing consolidation with fibrosis causing 'carnified lung' (Fig. 9.11).

Damage and destruction of bronchial walls during bronchopneumonic infections, particularly in childhood, can result in bronchiectasis and continuing symptoms and problems throughout life.

ASPERGILLOMA AS A LATE COMPLICATION

An aspergilloma can develop as a late complication in a residual lung cavity or cyst. Most usually this occurs in an old tuberculous upper lobe cavity but it is also seen on occasions associated with bronchiectasis, and post-pneumonic lung cavities. Colonization initially occurs on the wall of the cavity but, as time goes on, layers of necrotic debris and aspergillus peel off and form a mobile 'fungus ball' (Figs 9.14, 9.15 and 9.16). Haemoptysis is the major complication.

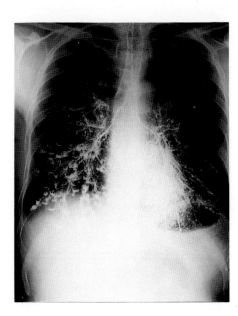

Fig. 9.12 This is a bronchogram of a 45-year-old man with a history of recurrent chest infections and daily cough and purulent sputum production for many years. He gave a history of 'double pneumonia' and pleurisy as a child. The changes of extensive cystic bronchiectasis can be seen in the right lower lobe, presumably as a consequence of childhood pneumonia.

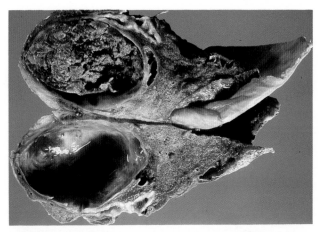

Fig. 9.14   A section of lung showing the appearance of a mycetoma within a cavity.

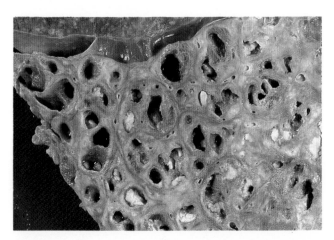

Fig. 9.13 In this example of an advanced stage of lower lobe cystic bronchiectasis following childhood pneumonia the lung parenchyma has been completely destroyed and replaced with pus-filled dilated thick-walled bronchi.

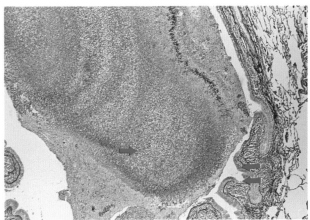

Fig. 9.15   A close view shows the ball of fungal hyphae (arrow) in the lumen of a respiratory epithelium lined sac (two arrows).

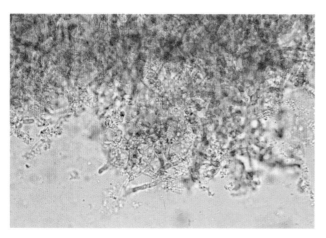

Fig. 9.16 The fungal ball can be seen to be made up of a tangle of fungal hyphae under high power magnification.

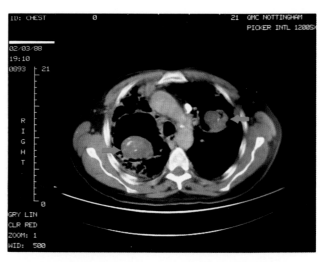

Fig. 9.18 Chest CT scan confirmed the aspergillomas bilaterally (arrowed) within large cavities. They had fallen to the dependent position within the cavities when the patient was lying on his back for the scan.

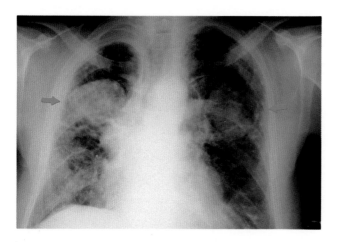

Fig. 9.17 A 60-year-old man had suffered from bronchiectasis following tuberculosis as a teenager. More recently he had had repeated haemoptysis. The chest radiograph showed bilateral aspergillomas (arrowed). The characteristic air crescents surrounding the aspergillomas are well seen.

FURTHER READING

Barker, A. F. and Bardana, E. J. (1988) Bronchiectasis – update of an orphan disease. *American Review of Respiratory Disease*, **137**, 969–77.

Muskett, A., Burton, N. A., Karwande, S. V. and Collins, M. P. (1988) Management of refractory empyema with early decortication. *American Journal of Surgery*, **156**, 529–32.

Sadigh, M. and Wassef, W. (1990) Parapneumonic effusions and empyema. *Current Options in Infectious Diseases*, **3**, 189–94.

10. Causes of Recurrent Respiratory Infections

If a patient suffers two or more episodes of pneumonia, an underlying reason should be suspected. If it recurs in one particular part of the lung a local structural problem is likely, whereas a more generalized disorder is possible when it recurs in different sites.

For localized recurrent infections a bronchial abnormality is possible, such as bronchial stenosis, bronchial obstruction, e.g. tumour or foreign body, or localized bronchiectasis, or pulmonary causes, such as sequestration, an area of organized pneumonia or lung fibrosis.

With recurrent non-localized pneumonia, general abnormalities of the lung are possible, including generalized bronchiectasis, cystic fibrosis, primary ciliary dyskinesia or chronic bronchitis. Of non-respiratory causes, silent aspiration is possible as a result of chronic sinusitis and postnasal drip, poor dental hygiene and caries, and oesophageal, neuromuscular or swallowing problems. Immune deficiency states must also be considered.

LOCALIZED CAUSES OF RECURRENT INFECTIONS

Examples of this are illustrated in the following case reports.

Bronchial obstruction

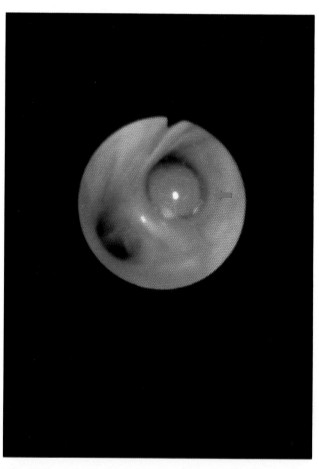

Fig. 10.2 At bronchoscopy, a smooth tumour was seen obstructing the right lower lobe bronchus (arrow).

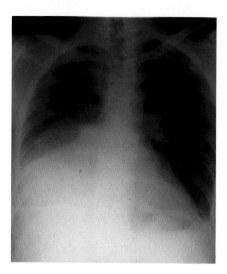

Fig. 10.1 A 26-year-old man was admitted to hospital as an emergency with right-sided pneumonia. He gave a history of several episodes of chest infection and 'pleurisy' on the right side over the previous five years. Chest radiography revealed right lower lobe collapse and consolidation.

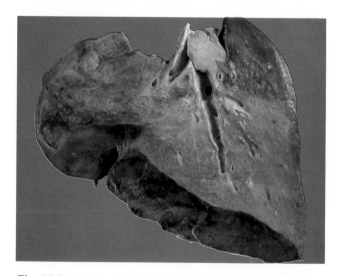

Fig. 10.3 At operation a large bronchial carcinoid tumour was found (one arrow) obstructing the right intermediate bronchus with a consolidation right lower lobe distally (two arrows) containing dilated bronchi. The right middle lobe was also involved.

Foreign body

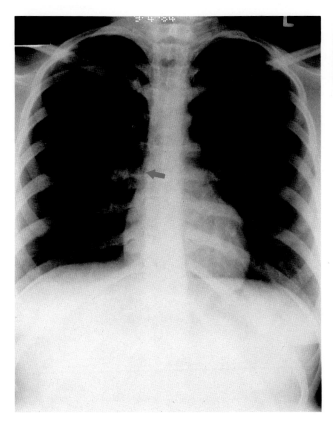

Fig. 10.4 A 13-year-old girl had recurrent chest infections for eight months. A wheeze was noted on the right side of her chest. The chest radiograph revealed an increased density at the right lower hilum (arrow).

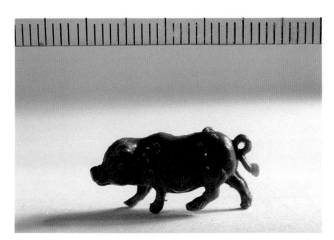

Fig. 10.5 A plastic pig, probably from inside a Christmas cracker, was extracted with difficulty from the right lower lobe bronchus at rigid bronchoscopy.

Bronchial stenosis

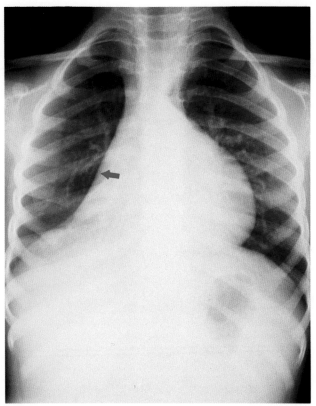

Fig. 10.6 A six-year-old Asian girl had been treated for tuberculosis of hilar glands two years previously and had since suffered from recurrent productive cough and respiratory infections. Flexible bronchoscopy showed a stenosis at the origin of the right middle and lower lobes, explaining the collapse (arrow) revealed on the chest radiograph. Some improvement following local bronchial dilatation.

Lobar sequestration

The term sequestration describes a developmental abnormality where a segment or lobe has abnormal bronchial and vascular communications to the rest of the lung. Intrapulmonary sequestrations are by far the commonest, usually occurring in the left posterior basal segment. Intrapulmonary sequestrations are usually silent in early childhood, presenting later with recurrent infections or haemoptysis. Surgical resection of a symptomatic segment is curative but trouble must be taken to identify the abnormal arterial supply preoperatively to prevent unexpected perioperative complications.

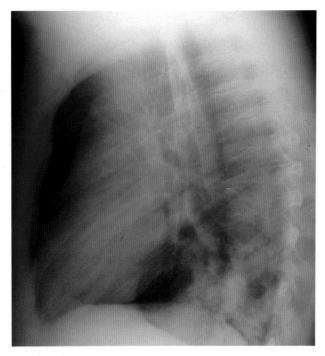

Fig. 10.7 Recurrent left lower lobe pneumonia was a clue to a local bronchopulmonary structural problem in an 18-year-old man.

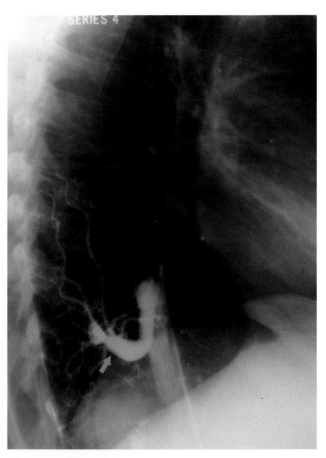

Fig. 10.9 An aortogram was performed which confirmed the diagnosis of lobar sequestration with aberrant arterial supply from the lower thoracic aorta (arrow). The sequestration was resected successfully with a partial lobectomy.

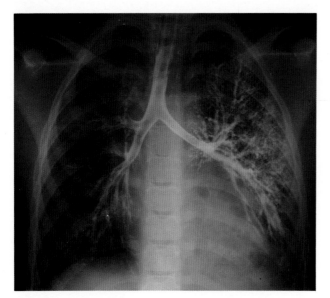

Fig. 10.8 A bronchogram revealed no bronchial connection to the left lower lobe basal segments.

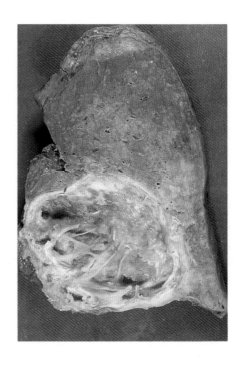

Fig. 10.10 A whole lung specimen from another case shows the features of a chronically infected and multi-cystic sequestration in the right lower lobe.

Bronchiectasis

Bronchiectasis is a common cause of recurrent respiratory infections and pneumonia.

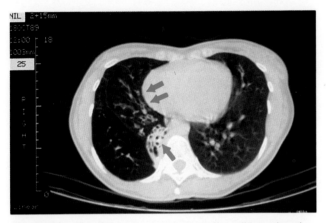

Fig. 10.11 This CT scan reveals a totally collapsed and bronchiectatic right lower lobe (one arrow) but also dilated, thickened bronchi in the right middle lobe (two arrows) and less so in the lingular. The patient, a 42-year-old housewife, was troubled by recurrent infections and chronic daily sputum production. Her symptoms were palliated but not cured by right lower lobectomy.

Fig. 10.12 Post mortem whole lung section of an elderly man who died of recurrent bronchopneumonia revealing gross upper lobe bronchiectasis but also large bronchiectatic bronchi in the lower lobe (arrow). Marked reaction pleural thickening present (double arrow).

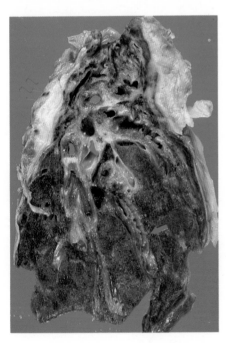

GENERALIZED RESPIRATORY CAUSES FOR RECURRENT INFECTION

Cystic fibrosis

Introduction

Cystic fibrosis is the commonest of the fatal inherited diseases in the white population and is characterized by the triad of chronic bronchopulmonary disease, pancreatic insufficiency and abnormal electrolytes in sweat.

In the last few years there have been enormous strides in the understanding of the genetic defect and the management of the condition such that now a median survival of 25–30 years is not uncommon. Currently there are at least 40 000 patients alive in Europe and the United States. By the year 2000, it is estimated that there will be over 6000 patients in England and Wales alone, 2600 of whom will be over 16.

Genetics and cloning the gene

This recessive genetic disease has a carrier frequency of about 1 in 25. The most well known and characteristic physiological defect is in chloride ion transport in secretory epthilelial cells.

Collaborative genetic work has led to the molecular cloning of the gene mutation responsible for the abnormal cystic fibrosis transmembrane regulation protein. A major mutation involving a three base pair loss at residue ΔF508 accounts for 70% or more of cystic fibroses mutations in Europe and North America. At least 60 other, less common, mutations have been described.

This discovery has opened up new avenues for screening and for gene-derived therapy. Gene transfer to cystic fibrosis cell lines with a retroviral vector is being explored.

Pathophysiology

The basic defect allows bacterial colonization of the respiratory tract, perhaps by facilitating bacterial adherence. This results in repeated episodes of infection. Widespread and progressive airways obstruction develops, with pulmonary tissue being affected only late in the disease. Immune function is probably largely normal and indeed chronic immune stimulation may itself contribute to tissue damage and progressive pulmonary dysfunction.

The pathological changes are those of chronic airways damage with bronchiectasis, and relative sparing of the alveoli.

In addition, changes invariably occur in the pancreas and liver.

Clinical features

In children, the condition can present as meconium ileus, failure to thrive and, most commonly, recurrent sinopulmonary infections.

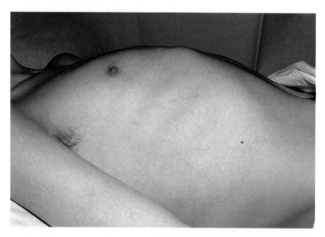

Fig. 10.13   Lateral photograph of a young adult with cystic fibrosis, demonstrating the barrel-shaped chest. Respiratory disease in CF adults is almost universal, with chronic cough and sputum production, haemoptysis, wheeze and subsequently chronic dyspnoea. In later stages, hypoxaemia leads to pulmonary hypertension and cor pulmonale. The majority of patients have finger clubbing and develop barrel-shaped chests due to airway narrowing, air trapping and hyperinflation.

Diagnosis and investigations

The sweat test remains the standard diagnostic test and in experienced hands is very reliable in children. It can be less reliable in adults unless a fluorohydrocortisone suppression test is included (Figs 10.14 and 10.15).

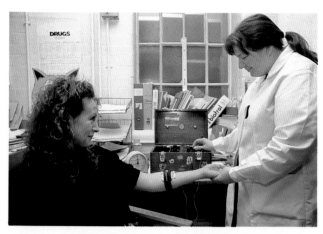

Fig. 10.14   A sweat test being performed using the Gibson and Cook method. Sweating is induced by pilocarpine iontophoresis. The weak current applied for 5 min aids penetration of the pilocarpine into the skin.

Fig. 10.15   The sweat is absorbed onto preweighed filter paper firmly attached to the skin for 30 min. Once over 100 g of sweat has been collected, this is eluted and the sodium and chloride concentrations measured by flame photometry. CF children have sweat sodium and chloride levels in excess of 60 and 70 mmol/litre respectively. If the result is equivocal in adults, oral fludrocortisone can be taken for two days; this will cause electroloyte suppression in the normal, but not CF, individual.

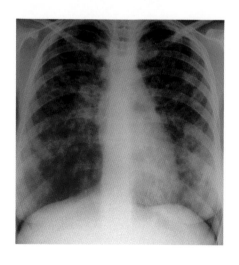

Fig. 10.16   The chest radiograph of a young adult with advanced cystic fibrosis showing hyperinflated lung fields and scattered proximal patchy consolidation. The initial changes on the chest radiograph include upper zone bronchial wall thickening. Fluffy nodular shadows, scattered atalectasis, hyperinflation and enlargement of the right heart and pulmonary arteries are seen as the disease progresses.

Microbiology

The bacteria usually isolated from the sputum of adults are *Pseudomonas aeruginosa* (83%) (Fig. 10.17), *Haemophilus influenzae* (68%) and *Staphylococcus aureus* (60%). The latter is usually the first pathogen to be isolated from children.

More recently another *Pseudomonas* species, *Ps. cepacia*, has been associated with rapid deterioration in some patients.

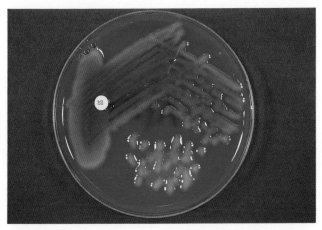

Fig. 10.17 ***Pseudomonas aeruginosa* grown on a blood agar plate.** This was a sputum isolate from a 16-year-old girl with advanced cystic fibrosis and shows a typical mucoid appearance. It was found to be resistant to ceftozidime but sensitive to imipenem and tobramycin.

Case history

Fig. 10.18 This chest radiograph is of a 22-year-old girl with cystic fibrosis who developed *Pseudomonas cepacia* infection. Compared with her chest radiograph taken three months earlier (see Fig. 10.16), there has been a dramatic deterioration. The organism was resistant to most antibiotics apart from ceftazidime and her condition rapidly deteriorated.

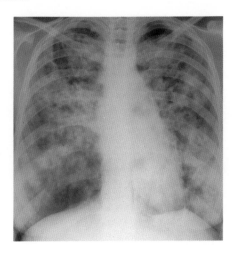

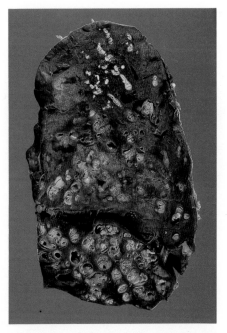

Fig. 10.19 At post mortem the lung showed cystic dilatation of the air passages with these bronchiectatic 'cysts' being filled with purulent material.

Management

Good nutrition and regular chest physiotherapy (Figs 10.20 and 10.21 are) essential in the overall management plan. Bronchodilators and on occasions inhaled corticosteroids are often beneficial.

Infections with *H. influenzae* and *Staph. aureus* can be treated with oral antibiotics, but the majority of adults are chronically colonized with *Ps. aeruginosa*, which requires intravenous antibiotic therapy. Usually two synergistic antibiotics are given, such as aminoglycoside (gentamicin, tobramycin) together with a carboxypenicillin (ticarcillin, carbenicillin) or an ureidopenicillin (azlocillin, mezlocillin, piperacillin) or a third generation cephalosporin (ceftazidime). Sensitivity testing and cost dictate the choice).

Intravenous therapy for the treatment of exacerbations is normally given for at least 10 days and some patients may learn to give their own antibiotics at home either via a peripheral long line (Fig. 10.22) or a Port-a-cath implanted in the chest wall to provide easy venous access (Fig. 10.23).

Orally active quinolones, such as ciprofloxacin, are now widely used for exacerbations, are very effective and are more convenient. The possible emergence of drug-resistant organisms remains a concern.

Ps. cepacia can be a particular problem as many organisms are resistant to most drugs.

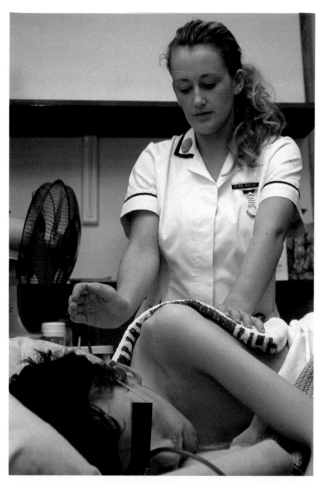

Fig. 10.20   Percussion physiotherapy and drainage is an essential part of management of the respiratory complications of cystic fibrosis.

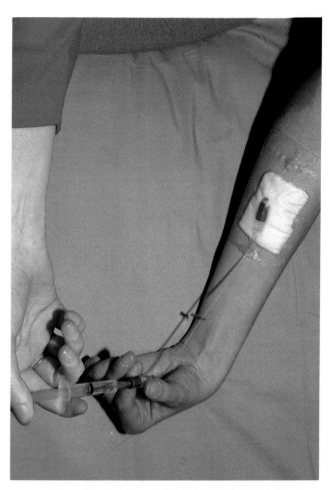

Fig. 10.22   This 18-year-old cystic fibrosis patient is learning to give his own antibiotic therapy through an intravenous long line inserted in his left forearm.

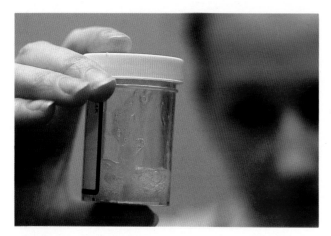

Fig. 10.21   Physiotherapy is effective at promoting sputum expectoration. Note the green colour of the sputum from *Pseudomonas aeruginosa* infection.

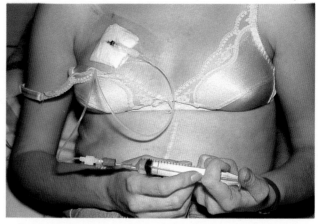

Fig. 10.23   This young patient is able to give her own intravenous therapy through an implanted venous access device on her chest wall. Devices such as Port-a-cath provide long-term, easy venous access.

Nebulized antibiotics, given twice daily, have been shown to be beneficial in some patients requiring frequent hospital admissions or who have rapidly deteriorating lung function.

Other causes of recurrent infections

Although cystic fibrosis is the commonest congenital cause of recurrent respiratory infections, less common causes are sometimes seen.

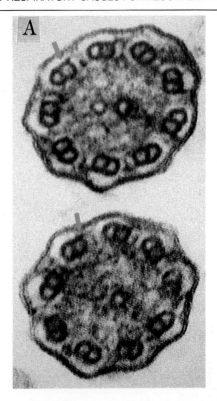

Fig. 10.26 A diagnosis of Katagener's syndrome or primary ciliary dyskinesia was made by examination of her nasal cilia. An elctro micrograph of a cross-section of two of her nasal cilia revealed absent or rudimentary inner dynein arms and short outer dynein arms (arrow).

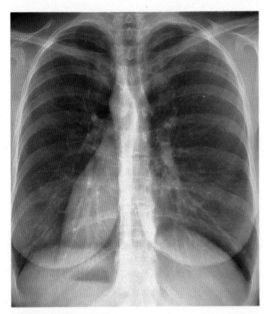

Fig. 10.24 A 20-year-old girl with the symptoms of bronchiectasis has dextrocardia and situs inversus well demonstrated on the chest radiograph.

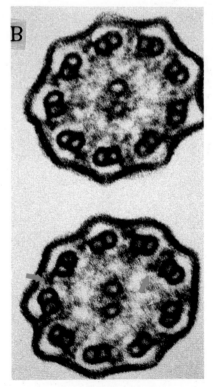

Fig. 10.27 In contrast a cross-section of normal cilia shows more obvious inner and outer dynein arms (arrow).

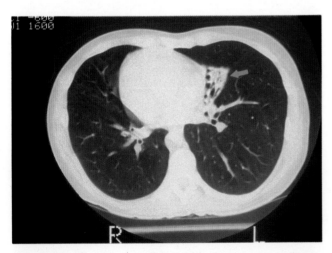

Fig. 10.25 Her CT scan of the chest shows some collapse and also bronchiectasis, particularly in her left middle lobe (arrow).

Primary ciliary dyskinesia is probably an autosomal recessive condition involving a disordered ciliary structure giving rise to poor ciliary function. There is partial or complete deficiency of outer or inner dynein arms which are responsible for powering ciliary action. Dextrocardia or situs inversus are present in about 50% of cases. Inefficient ciliary actions leads to generalized bronchiectasis, nasal disorders and problems with fertility.

NON-RESPIRATORY CAUSES OF RECURRENT INFECTIONS

Recurrent aspiration

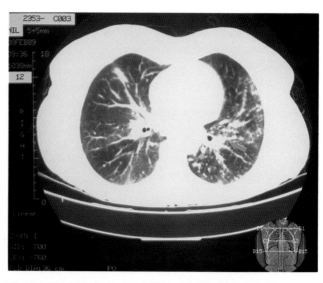

Fig. 10.29 This is a chest CT scan of a 50-year-old woman who complained of repeated attacks of noctural cough and also bronchitis at night. Scattered areas of consolidation and fibrotic lines are seen, particularly in the left lung (arrow).

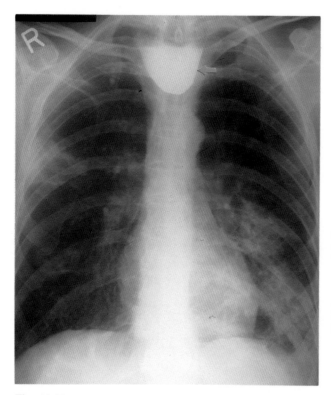

Fig. 10.28 An elderly patient had complained of recurrent cough after food and repeated chest infections. He was admitted with acute bilateral pneumonia. During recovery a barium swallow revealed a large pharyngeal pouch (arrow). The pouch was removed surgically and he had no further episodes of pneumonia.

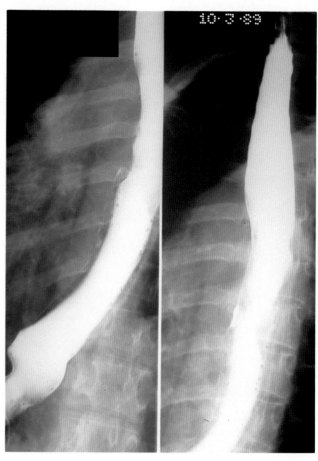

Fig. 10.30 Although she gave no history of oesophageal symptoms, a barium meal revealed free gastro-oesophageal reflux in the supine position with silent aspiration on screening. Her symptoms resolved after gastric fundoplication.

Other examples of aspiration-related pneumonia are discussed in Chapter 7.

Chronic sinusitis

Chronic sinusitis can sometimes cause recurrent lower respiratory infections due to postnasal drip and aspiration of infected material, probably mainly at night (Fig. 10.31; see also Chapter 3).

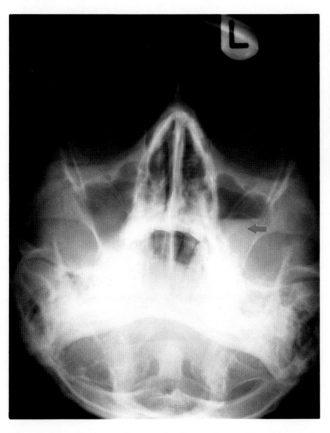

Fig. 10.31 Sinus radiograph of a patient with recurrent respiratory infections. The left maxillary sinus contains a fluid level (arrow) and the right is opaque.

Generalized non-respiratory causes of recurrent infection

Congenital or acquired immune deficiency should always be considered in patients of any age with recurrent pneumonia. Immunoglobulin levels should be checked in such cases, including IgG subclasses where appropriate. Replacement intravenous gammaglobulin therapy can transform the lives of such patients by reducing the burden of recurrent chest infections.

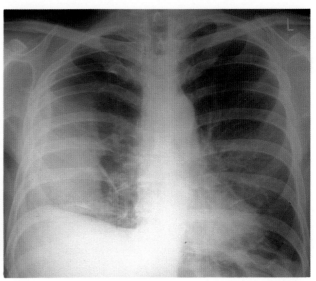

Fig. 10.32 A 60-year-old man presented with his second episode of bacterial pneumonia within 18 months. On this occasion it was complicated by a right-sided pneumococcal empyema. Investigations revealed hypogammaglobulinaemia associated with a thymoma that was surgically excised. He has continued to require gammaglobulin replacement therapy.

FURTHER READING

Abrutyn, E. (1984) Recurrent pneumonia. In *The Pneumonias* (ed. M. E. Levison), pp. 153–66. Wright PSG, Massachusetts.

Geddes, D. M., Warner, J. O. and Hodson, M. E. (1990) Cystic fibrosis. In *Respiratory Medicine* (eds R. A. L. Brewis, G. J. Gibson and D. M. Geddes), pp. 760–89. Baillière Tindall, London.

Hoiby, N. and Koch, C. (1990) *Pseudomonas aeruginosa* infection in cystic fibrosis and its management. *Thorax*, **45**, 881–4. (Note: this is one in a series of excellent review articles on cystic fibrosis in *Thorax* in 1990 and 1991.)

Kaltreider, H. B. (1986) Immune defences of the lung. In *Respiratory Infections* (eds M. A. Sande, L. D. Hudson and R. K. Root), pp. 47–70. *Contemporary Issues in Infectious Diseases*, vol. 5, Churchill Livingstone, New York.

11. Mycobacterial Infections

Mycobacterial infections can be divided into tuberculosis and those caused by non-tuberculous mcyobacteria.

TUBERCULOSIS

Tuberculosis continues to be a major world health problem. Although available statistics suggest a worldwide reduction in the incidence of tuberculosis, this must be viewed with caution as reporting may not be adequate in developing countries where tuberculosis is still rife.

In the Western world until recently, there had been a progressive annual decline in the number of new cases of around 7% per year. However, since 1986 in the United States and 1988 in Britain, there has been a small rise in the number of reported cases, ascribed to the occurrence of tuberculosis amongst patients with HIV disease. Tuberculosis is the commonest presentation and cause of death from HIV disease in Africa.

In England and Wales notifications have fallen from 7406 in 1982 to 5432 in 1989 with 443 deaths in 1989. This decline has disappeared in the last three years and is a cause for concern.

Pathogenesis

Mycobacterium tuberculosis is transmitted by infected droplets from an untreated patient with pulmonary tuberculosis. Initial infection usually involves a very localized, asymptomatic and self-limiting area of pneumonic inflammation followed a few weeks later by cell-mediated immunity to the tuberculin antigen, which results in the development of granulomas or 'tubercles'. In most cases the activated macrophages (epithelioid cells) will arrest bacillary growth and either kill off the bacteria or encapsulate them at the site of primary infection, although lymph node involvement is usual. Disease occurs when either the site of primary infection progresses by direct extension or there is spread by the lymphatics or the bloodstream. This can occur in young people during the first two years of initial infection or by secondary endogenous reactivation of a tubercle later in life when host defences are reduced for some reason. This latter mechanism is by far the commonest cause of new cases of tuberculous disease.

Clinical features in children

Primary infection is normally asymptomatic, being only discovered by the development of tuberculin sensitivity or the discovery of an old calcified primary focus on routine chest radiograph. In children, if a primary infection progresses, disease can be associated either with spread to the mediastinal lymph nodes or via the bloodstream to produce a miliary pattern sometimes complicated by meningitis. These are illustrated in Figs 11.1–11.3.

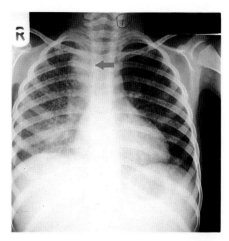

Fig. 11.1 Miliary tuberculosis with associated upper mediastinal lymphadenopathy (arrow) in a child who presented with tuberculous meningitis. His father was found to be the source case on contact tracing.

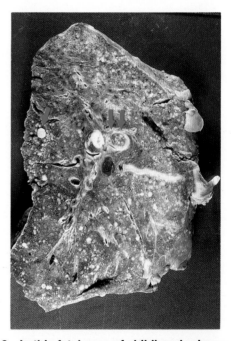

Fig. 11.2 In this fatal case of childhood primary tuberculosis there is a circumscribed caseous focus of primary infection (arrow) in the upper lobe with spread of the infection to caseating hilar lymph nodes (two arrows) and numerous blood-borne miliary tubercles in the rest of the lung.

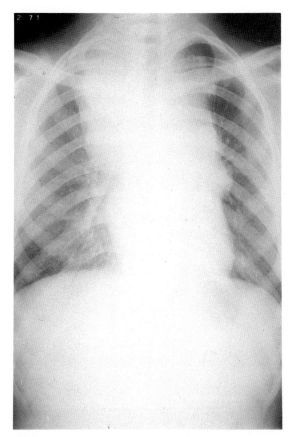

Fig. 11.3 This chest radiograph shows massive mediastinal lymphadenopathy without an obvious primary focus in the lung which is presumably too small to be seen. Tuberculosis was diagnosed by biopsy via a mediastinoscope in this teenage Asian girl.

Clinical features in adults

The classical presentation of pulmonary tuberculosis in an adult is with progressive weight loss, malaise, sweats, productive cough and haemoptysis.

The typical radiographic features of pulmonary tuberculosis arising from endogenous reactivation are consolidation and cavitation in one or both upper lobes (Fig. 11.4).

This is illustrated in the following case histories.

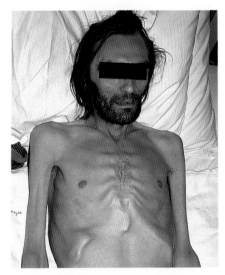

Fig. 11.5 This 48-year-old vagrant presented with marked cachexia, wasting, and cough and was found to have extensive sputum smear-positive pulmonary tuberculosis.

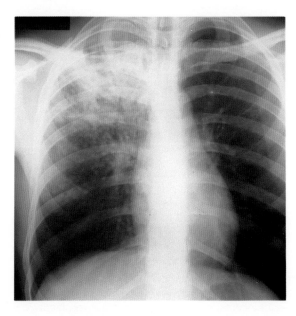

Fig. 11.4 Typical radiographic features of reactivated pulmonary tuberculosis.

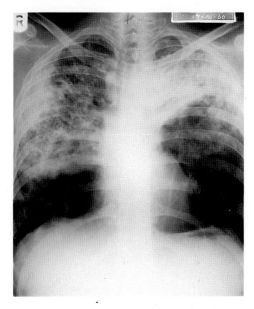

Fig. 11.6 His chest radiograph showed extensive and upper zone bilateral consolidation and cavitation.

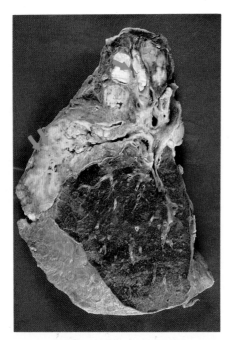

Fig. 11.7 In this fatal case of acute reactivation of tuberculosis in an elderly man, the apical areas of the upper lobe show chronic fibrocaseous disease (one arrow) with the lower segment showing acute caseous bronchopneumonia (two arrows).

An acute bronchopneumonic illness is less common but can occur is a caseous turbercle ruptures into a bronchus, producing bronchogenic spread as shown in Fig. 11.7 and the following case histories.

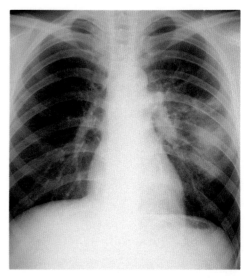

Fig. 11.9 A 19-year-old white man presented with a three week history of fever, malaise, and productive cough, and had patchy shadowing in the left lower lobe from acute tuberculous bronchopneumonia.

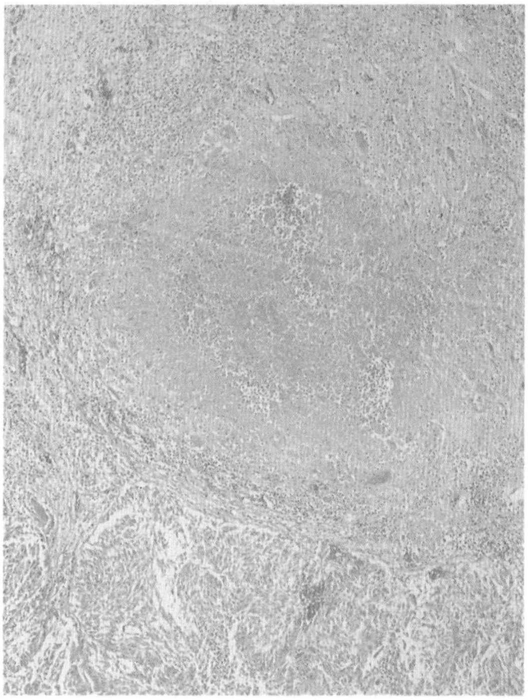

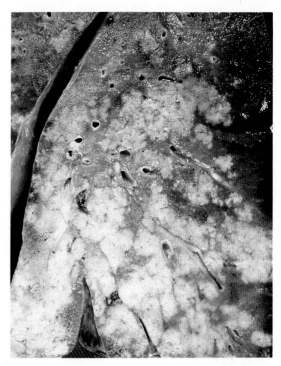

Fig. 11.8 Lung tissue from the same case (Fig. 11.7) showed the typical histological features of a tubercle with central caseous material and surrounding inflammatory reaction consisting of Langhans' multinucleate cells, epithelioid cells and lymphocytes.

Fig. 11.10 In this fatal case of acute tuberculous bronchopneumonia the lower lobes show confluent caseous pneumonic consolidation which emphasizes the lobular structure of the lung.

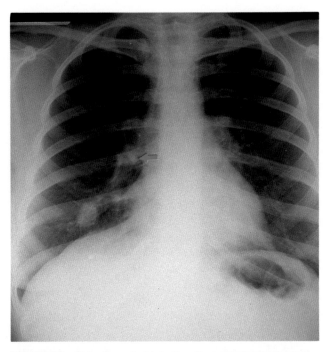

Fig. 11.11 This discrete high density mass in the right middle lobe was identified on a routine chest radiograph of a 40-year-old teacher applying for a job. Some calcification can also be seen in the region of the right hilar glands (arrow).

Fig. 11.12 The CT scan revealed a round lesion with a thick shell of calcification which was confirmed to be a 'tuberculoma' by excision biopsy.

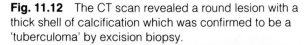

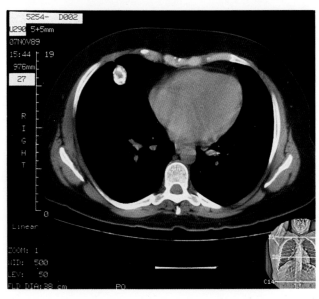

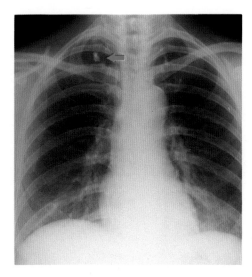

Fig. 11.13 This is another example of an 'old' calcified tuberculous focus found on routine chest radiograph (arrow). However, this 52-year-old woman was receiving immunosuppressive therapy following a renal transplant, had developed a productive cough and had positive sputum smears for *M. tuberculosis*. Immunosuppression had allowed the bacilli previously dormant in her apical primary focus to reactivate and cause disease with minimal pulmonary reaction.

Pleural involvement

Young adults can also present with tuberculous-related pleural effusions, usually when the infection has spread via the pulmonary lymphatics to involve the pleural surface.

Fig. 11.14 A 25-year-old white alcoholic male presented with a massive pleural effusion; the fluid was a straw-coloured exudate and the diagnosis of tuberculosis was made by histological examination and culture of pleural biopsies.

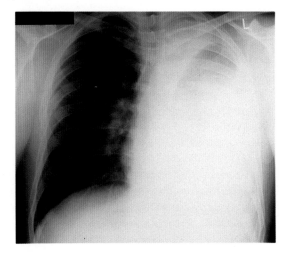

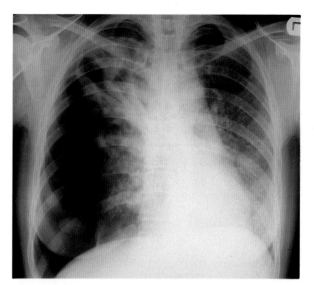

Fig. 11.15 Pleural involvement may also occur by rupture of a caseous lesion into the pleural space, resulting in an empyema or pyopneumothorax. This occurred in a 45-year-old woman who presented with acute dyspnoea following a six-week history of cough and weight loss.

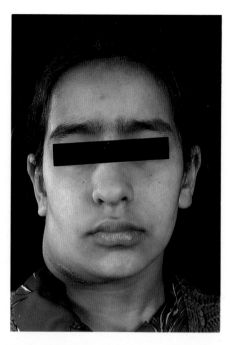

Fig. 11.17 Infection in non-pulmonary sites occurred in this 18-year-old Asian woman. The diagnosis was confirmed by lymph node biopsy. In young children cervical lymphadenopathy is not infrequently caused by atypical mycobacteria such as *Mycobacterium avium complex*, which histologically shows similar features.

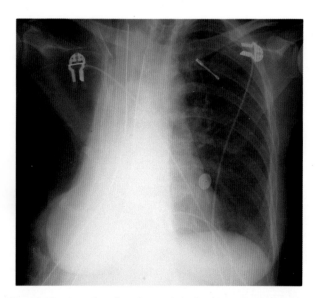

Fig. 11.16 In spite of prolonged drainage and appropriate anti-tuberculous chemotherapy, her infection did not settle and she required a pleuropneumonectomy and thoracoplasty.

Non-pulmonary tuberculosis

Extrapulmonary tuberculosis is commoner in those of Asian and African ancestry. In Britain, nearly half of Asian patients present with infection in non-pulmonary sites, the commonest being in cervical lymph nodes.

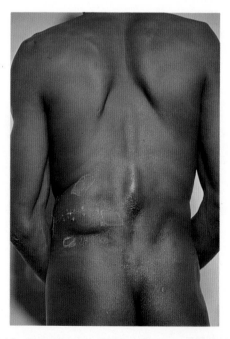

Fig. 11.18 This 40-year-old Nigerian presented with back pain for one month and a fluctant swelling in the left flank. Tubercle bacilli were identified in the pus aspirated from the cold abscess.

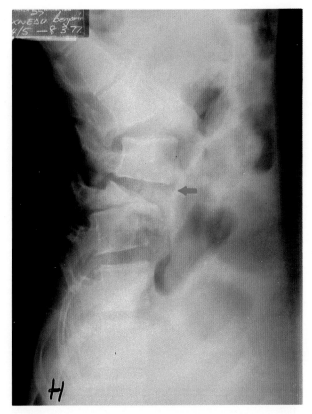

Fig. 11.19 His lateral spine radiograph at the level of the gibbus shows collapse of the second lumbar vertebrae and loss of disk space characteristic of infection (arrow). His chest radiograph showed some loss of volume and fibrotic shadowing in the right upper lobe suggestive of chronic pulmonary tuberculosis.

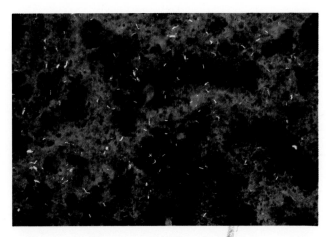

Fig. 11.20 Tubercle bacilli show up as brightly staining rods using fluorescent auramine stains.

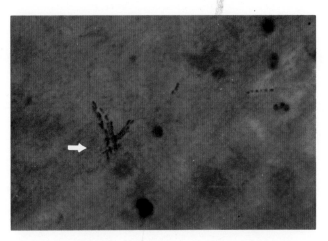

Fig. 11.21 Positive Ziehl-Neelsen stain of acid- and alcohol-fast bacilli. In this case, the long beaded appearance (arrow) is highly suggestive of *Mycobacterium kansasii*, the commonest of the pathogenic atypical mycobacteria.

Diagnosis of tuberculosis

Tuberculosis is most confidently diagnosed either by identification or culture of the organism or by a characteristic, clinical and histological presentation. Tuberculin reactivity can be a useful pointer to occult disease, particularly in children or other individuals, whom one would otherwise expect to be tuberculin negative. On occasions the diagnosis rests on a successful therapeutic trial of antituberculous chemotherapy in a patient with unexplained pyrexia or chronic illness.

Staining technique

Fluorescent auramine stains are frequently used for the rapid screening of specimens for tubercle bacilli, the organisms showing up as multiple, stained rod-shaped bacteria (Fig. 11.20).

Ziehl-Neelsen stain is used to positively confirm acid and alcohol fastness in bacilli (Fig. 11.21).

Tuberculin skin testing

This can be performed as a Heaf test, a Mantoux test or a tine test.

The Mantoux test has the advantage of delivering a precise amount of tuberculin and allowing more accurate grading of responses to different strengths. It requires some time and expertise to perform the correct intradermal injection and is less suitable for mass screening than the Heaf test. Figure 11.26 illustrates a strongly positive reaction to intradermal tuberculin (1:1000 strength) in a laboratory worker with occupational exposure to *Mycobacterium tuberculosis*.

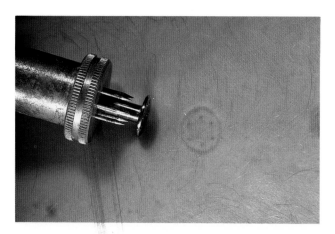

Fig. 11.22 A multiple puncture Heaf tubercilin skin test is being performed in this example. The six needles are fired though a film of tuberculin solution to a depth of 1–2 mm intradermally.

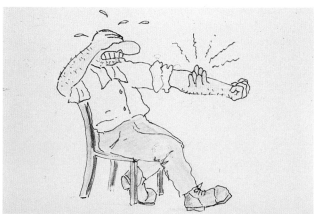

Fig. 11.25 This cartoon was drawn by a patient who developed a grade 4 Heaf test response, emphasizing that the test can be quite uncomfortable if strongly positive!

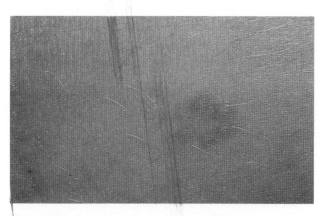

Fig. 11.23 The site is inspected 3–7 days later. In this case six papules are presented joined in a palpable ring – a grade 2 positive Heaf test suggesting some immunity.

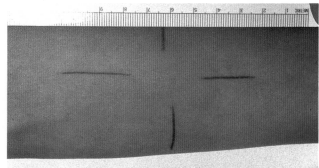

Fig. 11.26 **A strongly positive reaction to intradermal tuberculin (1 : 1000 strength) in a laboratory worker with occupational exposure to *M. tuberculous* (a positive Mantoux test).**

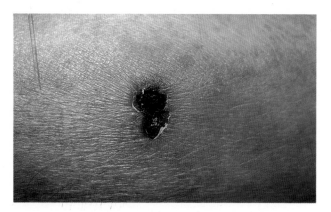

Fig. 11.24 In this case, an ulcerated grade 4 Heaf test has developed in a man subsequently diagnosed as having active pulmonary tuberculosis.

Management of tuberculosis

The mainstay of management is properly supervised, long-term therapy with combination antituberculous antibiotics. The most effective and commonly used antibiotics include rifampicin, isoniazid, pyrazinamide, ethambutol and streptomycin. Current recommendations for treatment vary from country to country.

The American Thoracic Society recommend a combination of isoniazid, rifampicin and pyrazinamide for the first two months followed by isoniazid and rifampicin for four months. The British Thoracic Society recommend the same drugs together with ethambutol for the first two months followed by isoniazid and rifampicin for four months. Without the initial ethambutol, continuation double therapy is recommended for up to seven months. On occasions more prolonged therapy is indicated and intermittent supervised therapy can be very effective where compliance is a problem.

With prolonged therapy, compliance can be a problem. A simple test of drug compliance is to look at urine colour. Rifampicin colours it pinky orange for 12–18 hours after dosage (Fig. 11.27).

The types and combinations of antituberculous antibiotics that can be used for treatment are many and therapy should be supervised by a physician experienced in their use (Fig. 11.28).

Disease prevention

In many countries there are active and successful BCG vaccination programmes which can give up to 80% protection against acquiring disease. In Britain BCG is offered to Asian babies at birth (due to their significantly increased incidence of tuberculosis), to other babies at birth where there is a near family history of tuberculosis, to Heaf-negative schoolchildren at age 13, and to non-immune contacts of cases of tuberculosis and workers at special risk of infection such as health care workers. The technique of BCG vaccination is illustrated below.

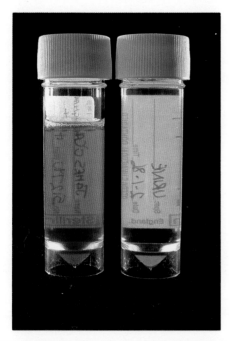

Fig. 11.27 The left-hand orangy sample of urine is from a patient on rifampicin compared with normal urine on the right.

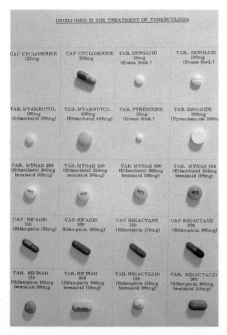

Fig. 11.28 An example of the many different strengths and combinations of antituberculosis antibiotics that are available.

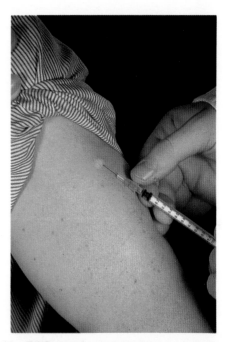

Fig. 11.29 BCG vaccine being given by intradermal injection. Intradermal BCG vaccination is normally given in the left upper outer forearm at the insertion of the deltoid muscle. Puckering and blanching of the skin confirms correct intradermal injection technique. Subcutaneous infections can result in abscess formation.

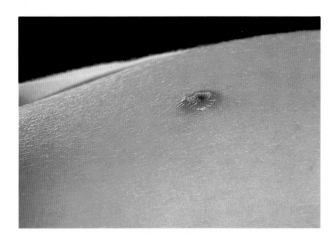

Fig. 11.30 Induration and inflammation appears at the site of a properly given BCG vaccination within 2–4 weeks.

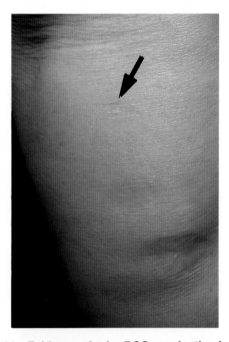

Fig. 11.31 Evidence of prior BCG vaccination is shown by a small pitted scar (arrow).

NON-TUBERCULOUS MYCOBACTERIA (ATYPICAL MYCOBACTERIA)

Non-tuberculous mycobacteria have assumed increasing importance over the last few years, firstly because of the importance of atypical mycobacteria such as *M. avium* complex in AIDS patients (see Chapter 6), and also with their increasing importance in percentage terms as a cause of pulmonary tuberculosis as the number of *M. tuberculosis* cases falls.

Classification

The classification is based more on laboratory features than differing clinical features, of which there are few. The classification take into account colony characteristics, pigment production on exposure to light and growth rate as illustrated in Table 11.1.

M. kansasii is the commonest non-tuberculous mycobacterium and is classified as a slow-growing photochromogen (Fig. 11.32).

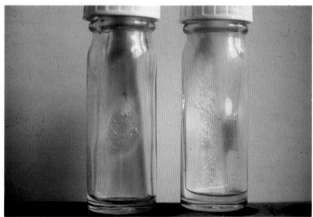

Fig. 11.32 Examples of *M. kansasii* growing on Lowenstein–Jensen medium. The culture on the left has been exposed to light which has encouraged the production of bright yellow carotene pigment in contrast to the culture on the right that has been kept in the dark.

M. fortuitum is an example of a rapid grower. Growth occurs within seven days of blood agar. Other acid-fast bacteria require 3–4 weeks to become well developed.

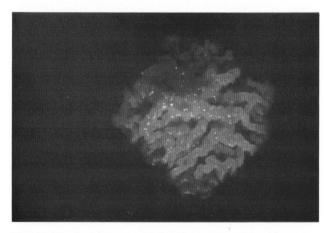

Fig. 11.33 In this case, *M. fortuitum* was cultured from the pus that discharged from enlarged cervical lymph nodes in a child with tuberculous lymphadenitis.

Table 11.1 Classification of non-tuberculous mycobacteria

Group	Characteristics	Growth rate	Species that are human pathogens
I. Photochromogens	Bright yellow–red, growth in light, not dark	Slow	*M. kansasii* *M. simiae* *M. marinum*
II. Scotochromogens	Yellow–orange, growth in light and dark	Slow	*M. xenopi*
III. Non-photochromogens	No colour	Slow	*M. avium* complex
IV. Rapid growers	Variable colour	Fast	*M. fortuitum* *M. chelonei*

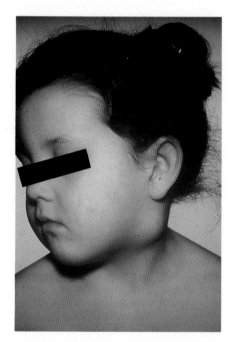

Fig. 11.34 The child had had painless lymphadenopathy for four weeks. The glands gradually settled without therapy.

Epidemiology

There is increasing awareness of disease caused by non-tuberculous mycobacteria as the incidence of disease caused by *M. tuberculosis* is falling. Probably 10–30% of all cases with mycobacterial disease now have non-tuberculous infection in Britain. It is uncertain how humans become infected with these environmental organisms and there is no good evidence for human to human transmission. The respiratory tract is presumed but not proven to be the portal of entry.

Pathogenesis

Generally these organisms have a low virulence and it is most likely that reduced host defences are important in allowing disease to develop. Many, but not all, patients have pre-existing chronic lung disease or some other factor affecting immune defences.

Clinical features

The presentation is similar to pulmonary tuberculosis except that the illness is more insiduous and generally the patient is less toxic. Underlying systemic or chronic pulmonary disease is common.

The chest radiograph can differ somewhat from pulmonary tuberculosis. Bronchopneumonia and pleural effusions are uncommon, coexisting chronic lung disease is usually apparent and thin-walled cavities with relatively little surrounding consolidation are said to be characteristic (Fig. 11.35).

Histologically the picture is similar to that seen in *M. tuberculosis* (Fig. 11.36).

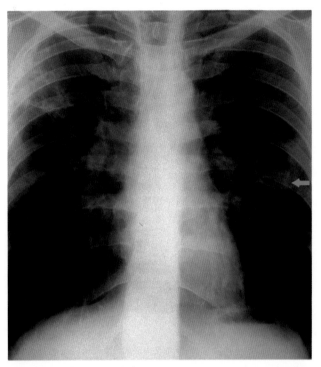

Fig. 11.35 Chest radiograph of a 45-year-old man with _M. kansasii_ infection. In addition to patchy consolidation, thin-walled cavities are present (arrow).

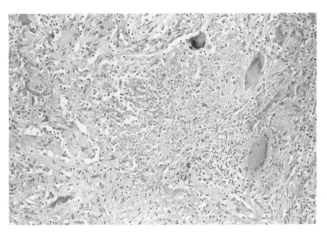

Fig. 11.36   In this case of _M. kansasii_ infection of the lung, there are poorly delineated giant cell granulomas with Langhans' giant cells but very few lymphocytes, suggesting an impaired immunological response to infection.

Management of atypical mycobacteria

The importance of these organisms is that they are usually resistant to one or more of the commonly used antituberculous antibiotics. For instance, _M. kansasii_ is invariably resistant to isoniazid and pyrazinamide and therapy requires prolonged treatment with rifampicin and ethambutol. More detailed discussion about therapy can be found in the sources quoted for further reading.

FURTHER READING

American Thoracic Society, Centers for Disease Control (1990) Diagnostic standards and classification of tuberculosis. _American Review of Respiratory Disease_, **142**, 725–35.

Joint Tuberculosis Committee of the British Thoracic Society (1990) Control and prevention of tuberculosis in Britain: an updated code of practice. _British Medical Journal_, **300**, 995–9.

Ormerod, L. P. (1990) Chemotherapy and management of tuberculosis in the United Kingdom: recommendations of the Joint Tuberculosis Committee of the British Thoracic Society. _Thorax_, **45**, 403–8.

Rieder, H. L., Cauthen, G. M. and Kelly, G. D. _et al._ (1989) Tuberculosis in the United States. _Journal of the American Medical Association_, **262**, 385–9.

12. Differential Diagnosis of Pneumonia (Mimics of Pneumonia)

When a diagnosis of pneumonia has been made but the patient does not improve as expected, a number of possibilities should be considered (Table 12.1).

In addition to these problems related to the pneumonia, the other possibility to consider is that the diagnosis of acute infective pneumonia is incorrect. A significant number of other conditions can mimic the clinical and radiographic features of acute pneumonia. Examples of some of these are given below.

PULMONARY INFARCTION

Not infrequently, pulmonary infarcts can present with fever, dyspnoea, cough, pleural pain, radiographic shadowing and neutrophilia in the blood.

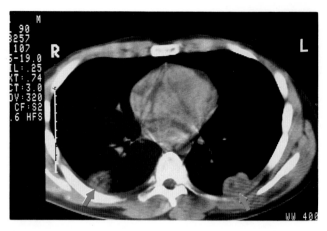

Fig. 12.2 A chest CT scan revealed bilateral cavitating subpleural shadows (arrows). Subsequent ventilation and perfusion isotope lung scans showed multiple unmatched defects with a high probability of pulmonary emboli. The patient made a complete recovery following anticoagulation.

Table 12.1 Factors to consider if a patient with pneumonia is responding slowly to therapy

Improvement expected too soon
Unexpected pathogen
Pathogen resistant to usual antibiotics
Local complication has developed, e.g. lung
    abscess, empyema
Distant complication, e.g. distant sepsis
Underlying bronchopulmonary disease, e.g.
    bronchial obstruction, bronchiectasis
Antibiotic hypersensitivity
Patient not receiving/taking treatment
Diagnosis of pneumonia is incorrect

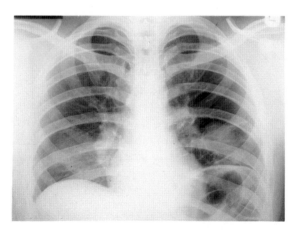

Fig. 12.1 This is the chest radiograph of a man who developed the above symptoms, including bilateral chest pain, eight days after an orthopaedic operation. Bilateral patchy shadowing is present which did not improve with antibiotic therapy.

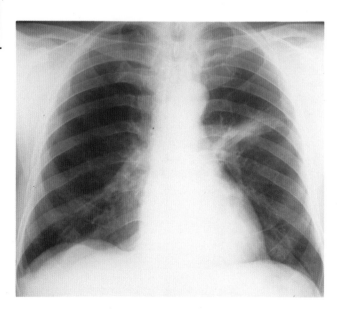

Fig. 12.3 As a contrast, another man developed similar symptoms a few days postoperatively and the chest radiograph shows left upper lobe segmental consolidation.

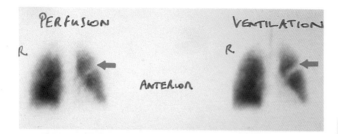

Fig. 12.4 A ventilation and perfusion isotope lung scan showed matched defects in the left upper zone (arrows) consistent with pneumonia and giving a low probability of pulmonary embolus. The patient improved with antibiotics. *Haemophilus influenzae* was cultured from his sputum sample.

A mixed clinical problem can develop when pulmonary infarcts become secondarily infected.

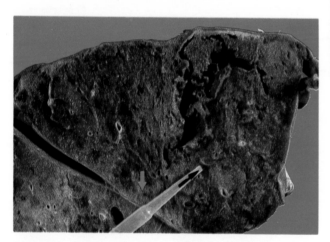

Fig. 12.5 A patient died of apparent cavitating bilateral basal pneumonia three weeks after hospital admission with a left hemiparesis. The section of lung shows a haemorrhagic focus due to an infected, cavitated pulmonary infarct. One of several emboli in the pulmonary arteries is identified by a pointer. Note the pale zone of demarcation of the infarct (arrow).

NON-INFECTIVE, INFLAMMATORY PNEUMONIAS

A number of inflammatory conditions can present with a history suggestive of infection and consolidation on the chest radiograph. Examples include eosinophilic pneumonia, bronchiolitis obliterans organizing pneumonitis (BOOP), vasculitis, particularly Wegener's granulomatosis, eosinophilic granu-loma and acute allergic or toxic alveolitis. Examples of some of these are given below.

Eosinophilic pneumonia

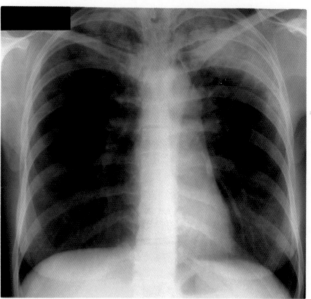

Fig. 12.6 Bilateral upper lobe consolidation is present on the chest radiograph of this 30-year-old woman who presented with fever, sweats, dry cough and dyspnoea which had not responded to two courses of antibiotics. Excess eosinophils were demonstrated both in peripheral blood and in bronchoalveolar lavage fluid, suggesting a diagnosis of eosinphilic pneumonia. She made a rapid recovery with oral corticosteroids. The dose of steroids was gradually reduced to zero over a two-month period with no evidence of relapse during prolonged follow-up.

Bronchopulmonary aspergillosis

Bronchopulmonary aspergillosis (BPA) is one form of pulmonary eosinophilia. The patient, often an asthmatic, develops a hypersensitivity to *Aspergillus* spp. This can result in recurrent episodes of bronchial and pulmonary inflammation presenting as attacks of bronchitis and bronchial plugging and/or flitting areas of lung consolidation. The clinical illness can mimic infection. Although eosinophils will predominate in the sputum and blood, *Aspergillus* may be cultured from bronchial secretions and *Aspergillus*-precipitating antibodies found in the serum.

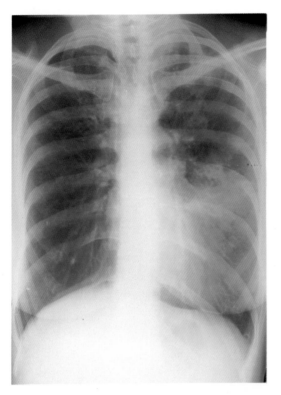

Fig. 12.7 A 50-year-old lady had first presented in 1974 with lingular 'pneumonia'.

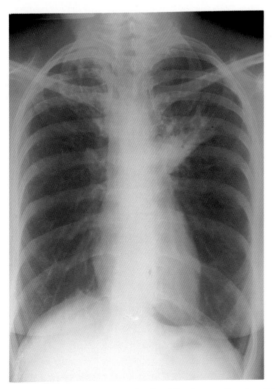

Fig. 12.8 Three years later she had had an episode of left upper lobe collapse and consolidation which had responded very slowly to antibiotics.

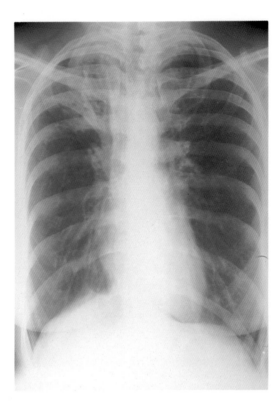

Fig. 12.9 It was only when she presented in 1986 with a similar illness affecting the right upper lobe that a diagnosis of BPA complicating her asthma was made. She improved with oral and inhaled corticosteroids.

On occasions, extensive mucous plugging can contribute to extensive lung collapse in BPA.

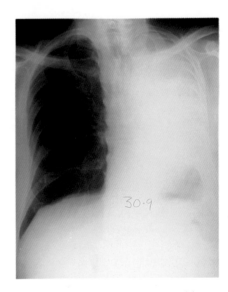

Fig. 12.10 Bronchoscopy on a 75-year-old man with left lung collapse and consolidation which had not improved with antibiotics revealed the left bronchial tree occluded by thick tenacious sputum.

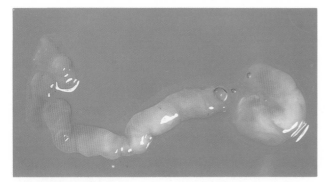

Fig. 12.11 Histological examination of a bronchial cast revealed abundant eosinophils and *Aspergillus fumigatus* was isolated on culture.

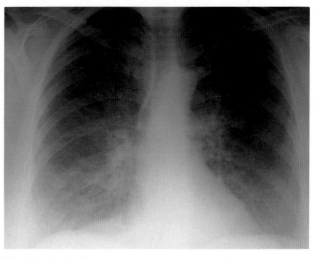

Fig. 12.13 A 50-year-old woman presented with dyspnoea, cough and fever for three weeks and consolidation in the right lower lobe.

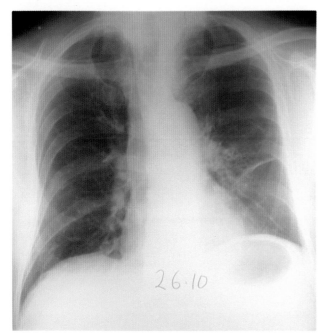

Fig. 12.12 Four weeks after starting corticosteroids, there was near complete re-expansion of the left lung. The patient had coughed up many sputum 'plugs'.

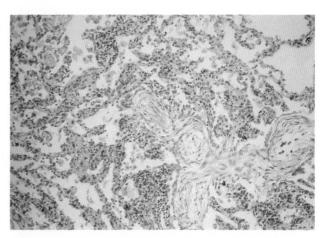

Fig. 12.14 Lung biopsy performed after no response to antibiotics revealed eosinophilic granuloma. The margin of a pulmonary nodule shows the extension of fibroblastic tissue as finger-like processes and the thickening of alveolar walls due to a pleomorphic cellular infiltrate.

Eosinophilic granuloma

Eosinphilic granuloma, now more properly called 'Langerhans cell granulomatosis', can also present subacutely with lung consolidation.

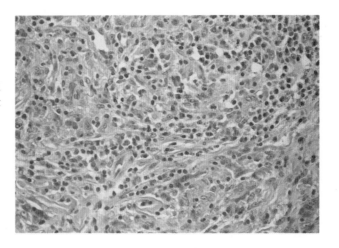

Fig. 12.15 (opposite) A higher power view shows a pleomorphic cellular infiltrate or large pale mononuclear Langerhans cells, lymphocytes and eosinophils, together with fibroblasts.

Bronchiolitis obliterans organizing pneumonitis

Pulmonary vasculitis

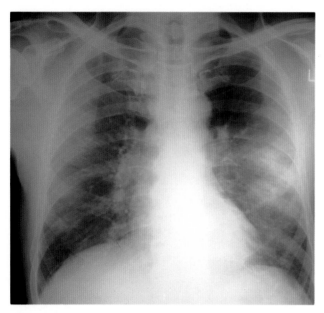

Fig. 12.16 In this case, open lung biopsy revealed that the consolidation in the left mid-zone of the lung was caused by bronchiolitis obliterans organizing pneumonitis (BOOP).

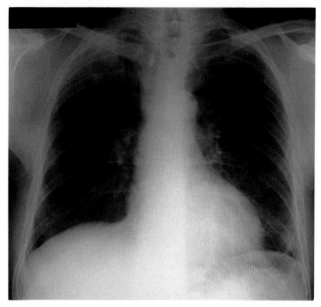

Fig. 12.18 Right upper lobe Wegener's granulomatosis consolidation can be seen on this chest radiograph of a 50-year-old man who presented with a three-week history of fever, night sweats, marked weight loss, malaise, nasal discharge, dyspnoea and dry cough.

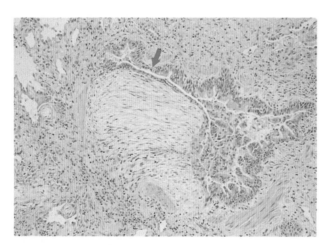

Fig. 12.17 The lung biopsy revealed a bronchiole (arrow) being eccentrically obliterated by young fibrous tissue forming in inflammatory areas. The patient had had a documented episode of right lower lobe consolidation three months previously almost certainly caused by the same condition. This condition responds well to corticosteroid therapy.

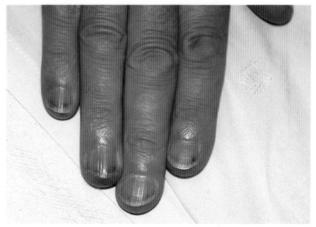

Fig. 12.19 One clue to the diagnosis in this case was the presence of nail bed vasculitic infarcts. The diagnosis was made by biopsy of an ulcer in the nose and evidence of renal involvement by crescentic glomerulonephritis. His symptoms and the lung consolidation cleared with intensive courses of cyclophosphamide and corticosteroids.

Allergic and toxic pneumonitis

A wide variety of drugs and chemicals either ingested or inhaled can produce an acute toxic or allergic pneumonitis. An unusual example is given below.

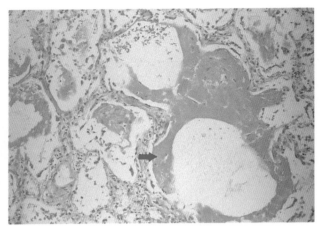

Fig. 12.22 He subsequently died and lung histology showed hyaline membranes lining the alveoli (arrow) which is typical of ARDS histologically.

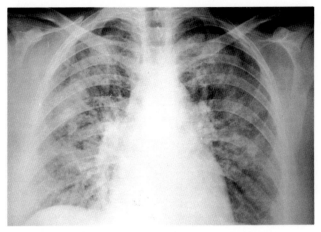

Fig. 12.20 A Spanish patient presented with acute fever, flu-like symptoms and 'pneumonia'. Very many cases occurred at the same time in Spain in 1981 and it was feared that a new type of infection had appeared. Eventually it was tracked back to an allergic or toxic reaction to the consumption of contaminated cooking oil producing a toxic pneumonitis.

MALIGNANT CONDITIONS MIMICKING PNEUMONIA

On occasions malignant conditions such as lymphoma or carcinoma, particularly alveolar cell carcinoma or metastatic lymphangitis carcinomatosis, can be confused with acute lung infections.

ACUTE RESPIRATORY DISTRESS SYNDROME – ARDS

A common problem on the intensive care unit is to differentiate infective lung shadowing from that of cardiogenic pulmonary oedema or ARDS.

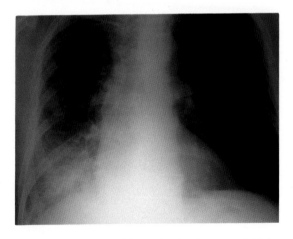

Fig. 12.23 A 79-year-old man had a three-week history of productive cough, fever and signs of the right base of the lung. There was no improvement with antibiotics, and transbronchial biopsy of the consolidation in the right lower lobe revealed alveolar cell carcinoma.

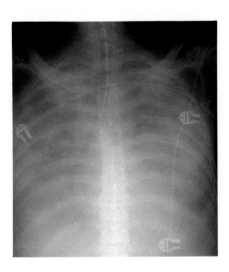

Fig. 12.21 (opposite) A 50-year-old man developed fatal ARDS following acute pancreatitis. Complete 'white out' of the lung fields is seen on the chest radiograph. There was no evidence of infection on bronchoalveolar lavage or protected specimen brush sampling.

FURTHER READING

Gibbs, A. R. and Anderson, E. G. (1990) Pulmonary vasculitis and eosinophilic pneumonia. In *Respiratory Medicine* (eds R. A. L. Brewis, G. J. Gibson, D. M. Geddes), pp. 1165–87, Baillière Tindall, London.

Index